VETERINARY PRACTICE MANAGEMENT SECRETS

VETERINARY PRACTICE MANAGEMENT SECRETS

THOMAS E. CATANZARO, DVM, MHA, FACHE
Diplomate, American College of Healthcare Executives
President and Chief Executive Officer
Veterinary Practice Consultants®
Golden, Colorado

PHILIP SEIBERT, JR., CVT
Consultant / Vice President for Support Services
Veterinary Practice Consultants®
Golden, Colorado

HANLEY & BELFUS, INC./ Philadelphia

Publisher: HANLEY & BELFUS, INC.
             Medical Publishers
             210 South 13th Street
             Philadelphia, PA 19107
             (215) 546-7293; 800-962-1892
             FAX (215) 790-9330
             Web site: http://www.hanleyandbelfus.com

Note to the reader: Although the information in this book has been carefully reviewed for correctness of dosage and indications, neither the authors nor the editor nor the publisher can accept any legal responsibility for any errors or omissions that may be made. Neither the publisher nor the editor makes any warranty, expressed or implied, with respect to the material contained herein. Before prescribing any drug, the reader must review the manufacturer's current product information (package inserts) for accepted indications, absolute dosage recommendations, and other information pertinent to the safe and effective use of the product described.

Library of Congress Cataloging-in-Publication Data

Veterinary practice management secrets / edited by Thomas E. Catanzaro, Philip Seibert, Jr.
        p. cm. — (The Secrets Series®)
     Includes bibliographical references and index.
     ISBN 1-56053-400-1 (alk. paper)
     1. Veterinary medicine—Practice.   I. Catanzaro, Thomas E.   II. Seibert, Philip, 1961–   III. Series.
SF756.4.V48   2000
636.089'068—dc21

00-023118

VETERINARY PRACTICE MANAGEMENT SECRETS   ISBN 1-56053-400-1

© 2000 by Hanley & Belfus, Inc. All rights reserved. No part of this book may be reproduced, reused, republished, or transmitted in any form, or stored in a data base or retrieval system, without written permission of the publisher.

Last digit is the print number: 9 8 7 6 5 4 3 2 1

CONTENTS

Preface v

Introduction 1

  1. Starting Your Practice 9
    Your New Clinic   9
    Location - Location - Location   12
    Financing Your Dream   14
    Leasehold Versus Free-Standing   15
    Budgeting   16
    Computerization   19
    Equipment and Inventory   29
    Safety Always!   30
    Early Staffing   31
    The Front Door Must Swing   35
    Marketing or Client Education?   36

  2. Human Resources 43
    Recruitment of the Right Staff   43
    Motivation Versus Incentives   45
    Creativity and Innovation   48
    Discipline Matters   51
    Policy Manuals   52
    Training Issues   53
    Setting Up the Schedule   55
    Millennium Management   56

  3. Staff Training and Orientation 61

  4. Regulatory Matters 71
    Health and Safety   71
    Controlled Substances   89
    Litigation Concerns   92

  5. Rights of the Employed 95
    Associates' Evaluation of Jobs   95
    Doctor Contracts   96
    Benefits Packages   97

  6. Ancillary Services 99
    Boarding   99
    Grooming   100
    Pet Boutiques and Photography   101
    Expanded Patient Services   102

7. Growing Beyond One Doctor 105
    Finding an Associate   105
    Work and Play Well With Others   106
    Expanding the Team   106
    Fees and Valuing Healthcare   110

8. Client/Customer Services (Smart Marketing) 113
    Client Versus Customer   113
    Longer Hours or Better Scheduling   113
    Price Shoppers   114
    Making the Front Door Swing   115
    Wellness Procedures   117
    Marketing Perspectives   121

9. Succession Planning 127
    Separation of Assets & Resources   127
    Slowing Down Your Life—Not Your Practice   128
    Passing On the Healthcare Team Leadership   128
    Retirement Concerns   129

10. And Then There Is Tomorrow 131
    Friends and Family Are Forever   131
    It's All In the Balance   132
    Efficacy, Efficiency, and Effectiveness   132

Appendix A 135
    Veterinary Management Sound Bites for Success

Appendix B 141
    Glossary of Terms

Appendix C 149
    Staff Training & Orientation Forms

Appendix D 159
    Reading List

Index 163

PREFACE

When asked by Hanley & Belfus, Inc. to write this Secrets text, we felt very complimented; they have published more than 45 well-respected books in The Secrets Series®. While Phil Seibert and I seldom *fully* agree on the best answer to a specific issue or challenge, and in some cases disagree on some of the alternatives in this text, we do concur that the diversity of this profession requires the wide spectrum of ideas that we have compiled.

We need to thank the members of the American Animal Hospital Association, the clients of Catanzaro & Associates, Inc., and the many practices sending inquiries into Veterinary Practice Consultants®. Without these 2400-plus practices, including the over 300 practices we support every year, the questions and answers would not have flowed.

The second group of folks we need to thank is our support team: Sylvia Zamperin, our new Client Relations Director, who ensures that our clients receive the most exacting of compassionate care; Courtney Edwards, our Communications Director, who assembled and grammar-proofed these submissions; Debbie Catanzaro, our Fiscal Director, who keeps our finances straight; Michael Catanzaro, our Continuing Education and Public Relations Director, who ensures that our multiple meetings and seminars stay coordinated and on track; and certainly our team of consultant associates (see them at our web site: www.v-p-c.com), who give us the freedom to share ideas and perspectives with the veterinary profession. We also must thank Karyn Gavzer, MBA, CVPM, a remarkable woman who we have known and admired for many years, for her contribution of 12 insightful marketing questions. Also, Judi Leake, DVM must be acknowledged for her continued support and vast knowledge of ancillary services.

Finally, we must thank our families, who not only help us stay balanced in life, but who endure many, many days and nights alone on the home front while we travel the world to pursue our chosen endeavors!

Thomas E. Catanzaro, DVM, MHA, FACHE
Philip Seibert, Jr, CVT

INTRODUCTION

As we were writing this practical reference, the American Veterinary Medical Association (AVMA), American Animal Hospital Association (AAHA), and American Association of Veterinary Medical Colleges (AAVMC) contracted a study of our profession and published a 23-page Executive Summary in JAVMA, Volume 215, No. 2, July 15, 1999. It is entitled, "The Current and Future Market for Veterinarians and the Veterinary Medical Services in the United States." The AVMA, AAHA, and AAVMC "mega-study" identified strengths and weaknesses of the veterinary profession as we enter the new millennium. The Summary is basically a list of problems: it provides no solutions. Hopefully, this text will stimulate veterinarians to seek new and innovative solutions to some old and stubborn problems.

The first secret in this text is: *Never blame!* When someone blames, they actually are abdicating accountability for resolution. It does not matter who or what you blame, it is a "cheap out" that does not improve the environment. We thought that a discussion of the study's **six critical issues** would make a wonderful introduction to this book, and illustrate the need for alternatives to cope with the dynamics of a changing environment. Since our premise is that no single best answer exists, and that there always are alternatives, we use these issues as a starting point to set the tone.

1. VETERINARIANS' INCOME

"The income of individual veterinarians seriously lags behind that of similar professions, and impacts the ability to repay student loans, to attract the best and brightest to the profession, and to invest in personal and professional growth. Further, pricing of veterinary services may not be appropriate relative to the real cost of the service and the value being delivered."

The study used terms like "similar professions" and "median income" to help set a base for comparison. To enhance the data, we would like to include human healthcare compensations for 1998: general practice physicians have an average income of $86,000; family practice specialists (boarded) have an average income of $132,000. These numbers are compatible with veterinary practice owner and specialty incomes. It appears that the $160,000 median physician salary used in the study comparisons included the "high-risk" specialties and ignored the liability and overhead costs of the human medical profession as compared to ours.

So, the good news is that the numbers are similar; therefore the real questions are: "Is this good enough?" and "What can we do to improve the numbers?" The role of the client-centered, patient-advocate provider is to **sell peace of mind**. This means offering two "yes" alternatives to meet the client's concern. It means bringing the pet back more often, not just raising the fee schedule to reduce the client's discretionary income to shock levels. This is called quality healthcare delivery and adds to the staff pride. Clients perceive pride as quality, and they are willing to pay for it in return for peace of mind.

We believe the answer to the first question is found in the belief of the individual practitioner. The answer to the second question is found in this book. (Especially see Chapters 6 and 7 for ideas on business expansion and income.)

2. ECONOMIC IMPACT OF LARGE NUMBERS OF WOMEN IN THE PROFESSION

"This study indicates that income of women veterinarians is seriously below that of their male colleagues. There is additional evidence that women work fewer hours, are less likely to be practice owners, and may price their services below that of men. There is a concern that these factors may be reducing the income levels of all veterinarians."

First, the sample appeared too small and not calibrated to the employment groups being compared. Most practices currently are owned by men that graduated two or more decades ago. Their compensation comes from clinical medicine, rental of building and land, and return on investment. Women are predominantly new entries into this profession and have only one source of income—clinical compensation. A stronger case can be made for income differences due to age differences rather than gender differences.

Second, most individuals 30 or younger—men *and* women—want a balanced life. New graduates are seeking outside-practice lifestyle development and a reasonable work week, not the 60–80 hours that past generations endured.

Third, hospital owners, not women associates, make price decisions. To blame reduced fee schedules on the new graduate is just one example of the old paradigms of the profession.

The real question may be: "What are we going to do with all these young women who are entering this profession?" The most obvious reply is to cherish their contributions and appreciate the compassionate care that they bring with them. Additionally, *everyone* deserves a quality of life in this profession that is better than what has gone before.

The breakthrough question this book attempts to answer is: "How can veterinary practices provide a good income and a reasonable work week?" In a multi-doctor practice, the new graduate and the seasoned veterinarian—men and women—can be "developed" into productivity-based veterinarians, supporting a high-density schedule and delivering quality veterinary healthcare. At 20% of personal productivity, most doctors can easily earn more than $50,000 a year on a 4-day work week and still get home for supper most evenings. (See Chapters 2, 4, and 6 for ideas and possible solutions.)

3. GLOBAL DEMAND FOR ALL CATEGORIES OF VETERINARY SERVICES

"While consumer (animal owner) spending on veterinary services has been robust, there is substantial opportunity to further increase demand. There also is evidence that there is a potentially significant market for veterinarians and veterinary services, particularly in nontraditional and nonprivate practice areas."

Millennium graduates have four to six job offers, and the AVMA Job Bank shows six to eight jobs for every applicant. These two reality factors were not included in any of the summarized research by this joint Committee, but these numbers strongly suggest a growing demand for both traditional and nontraditional veterinary services.

The study shows that client awareness and projected access should exceed the demand. We can assist practices in their effort to increase return rates. Higher return rates allow a practice to lower their fees, which in turn allows the clients who consider their pets members of the family to access more veterinary care within their available discretionary income levels. We can increase access virtually anywhere, from mixed animal to companion animal practices, if the cornerstone of the practice's healthcare delivery is **compassionate care** that celebrates the human-animal bond. (See Chapters 1, 5, and 7.)

4. INEFFICIENCY OF THE DELIVERY SYSTEM

"The majority of animal care is still being delivered through a highly fragmented and inefficient system. This includes issues related to excess capacity, staff utilization, and use of capital resources."

The linear scheduling promoted in most veterinary teaching hospitals (VTH) is appropriate for tertiary care facilities, but most general practices are primary care facilities and should be using **high-density scheduling**. A physician uses three to five consultation rooms and a larger nursing staff to move and screen clients. A dentist uses six to nine chairs and a skilled dental hygiene team to see 46–65 patients per day. These activities happen on time (more or less) and without overwhelming their system. Similar opportunities are available in veterinary practice.

Alternative veterinary healthcare delivery models exist, and have been published. The VTH and the traditional associations have not promoted these systems in their training, in their standards, or in their continuing education seminars. This study may be the "call to action" for those systems anchored in the past.

Another question to consider is: "How do we increase our effectiveness in delivery?" The answer is a basic and simple tenet. We must learn to use our nursing staff as well as the other healthcare professions have over the decades. Moreover, physician extenders, nurse practitioners, and a host of paraprofessional specialists, from anesthesiologists to physical therapists, can be brought to the practice. Yet many veterinarians seem to think they are the only ones in the practice with technical skills, so they must be the ones who "do it all." Veterinary practices that employ client-centered and patient-centered **veterinary extenders** as primary patient care providers and client relations specialists are already producing double to triple that of doctor-centered practices. (See Chapters 1, 6, and 7.)

5. SUPPLY OF VETERINARIANS

"There is evidence that, in purely economic terms, there is an excess of veterinarians, which is a cause of downward price pressure and is projected to result in stagnant veterinary incomes over the next 10 years. More important, the characteristics of the supply may not closely match the demand, and there is evidence that modifications in the education of veterinarians

will enable the profession to capitalize on emerging markets and to create new services."

"Downward price pressures" and "stagnant incomes" have little bearing on new graduates, or on the great shortage of veterinarians in private practice. We can place new graduates at $50,000 or more annual salary due to their demand. All we have to do is show practices how to use them for high-density scheduling, and they easily pay for their W-2 compensation.

One southeastern veterinary school had only 14 of their June 1999 graduates enter private companion animal practice; all others stayed in school, entered special interest areas, specialities, or stayed in the community waiting for their spouse to graduate.

The new graduate asks: "How can I prevent a stagnant income?" Practitioners ask: "How can any rational body of supposedly 'knowledgeable experts' say that there is an excess of veterinarians when there are so many jobs still unfilled?" Most observers agree that there is a mal-distribution of veterinarians, yet new graduates are so debt ridden that most will follow the highest pay offer outside of their geographic preference.

The reciprocal question for practice owners is: "What can I afford to pay an employed veterinarian?" The answer is, if a veterinary practice pays a doctor 20% of his or her personal examination, consultation, inpatient, and surgery production as compensation, in a practice with veterinary extenders, the owner can have as many associates as desired and continue to grow the practice's return on investment! Our job is to get the right doctor linked to the right practice at the right time. This need will likely generate veterinary-employee brokerages in the new millennium. (See Chapters 1, 2, 4, and 6.)

6. SKILLS, KNOWLEDGE, APTITUDE, AND ATTITUDE OF VETERINARIANS AND VETERINARY STUDENTS

"While there is ample evidence that the scientific and clinical skills of the profession remain very high, there is also evidence that veterinarians lack some of the skills and aptitudes that result in economic success. Additionally there is evidence that veterinarians' self perception of their abilities and their perception of what they can contribute to society potentially limit the profession and economic growth of the veterinary medical profession."

Most new graduates have never done a basic dental cleaning and polishing, much less an extraction; have not treated a cat fight abscess; and, in many cases, have not developed basic population control surgery skills. Yet the study states "clinical skills remain very high." As for "their perception of what they can contribute to society," neither the survey data nor our experience in this profession shows a lack of social contribution by the practitioners in a community. To the contrary, most practices support church, Rotary, civic organizations, and their community with time and money.

Here, the question is: "How do veterinarians get the business skills and aptitude to make their business successful?" The answer is obvious, yet seldom stated in this profession. Just buy them! Any practice owner can "buy" a banker, a good corporate attorney, a savvy CPA for tax reporting, and an ethical veterinary-specific consultant to form their business team. What most practices have done is buy the cheapest support available, and they have gotten what they paid for as well as a bucket of frustrations. If this profession's advisors/associations continue to think that a veterinarian can "do it all," then they do not understand the requirements of the business place. Financial planners are essential for developing a protected retirement fund—sorry, you cannot live off the practice sale anymore. Ethical consultants—ones who do not advocate deep-discount competition programs, or blindly push rapid fee increases, or take a portion of the growth as their compensation—are extremely beneficial when looking for alternatives (See Chapters 1–9.)

If the preceding text seems like a critically harsh evaluation of the Executive Summary of "The Current and Future Market for Veterinarians and the Veterinary Medical Services in the United States," it is only because we are asking our readers to see a different world than one full of problems. We want to provide alternatives for action, individually, by practice, and through established veterinary medical associations.
- We see most veterinarians supporting Rotary, school athletics, church, and other community functions. Veterinarians are some of the most educated professionals in their community, and often are members of various boards and committees.
- We see most veterinarians hindered by the traditional "chute mentality" taught to them in school and their earlier practices. One cow through a chute at a time means we schedule with one companion animal column per veterinarian on the appointment log.
- This survey uses the Canadian R. K. House & Associates, Ltd. 1992 survey and the *Anthrozoos* journal (Catanzaro is one of the few hundred subscribers to this Delta Society publication) for over 40% of their Executive Summary references, yet Pfizer has done significant practice and client research in the past few years (over 500 practices a

year). If we look at the Pfizer study data, alternatives leap forward and yell to be addressed, as they do in these chapters.
- We see some states severely restricting the role of the veterinary technician and nursing staff, while the human healthcare market embraces the physician extender. Yet association and university VTH experts do not address these fallacies and political misconceptions. Again, it is individual practitioners who must pick up the team approach and pursue success!
- We see many underpaid practice staffs because "We have always done it this way"; because "The national average says so"; or because "We center on expense control rather than income production." The key here is to accept the cost of a new staff replacement (> $23,000) and use that money to keep highly qualified staff members in this profession.
- We have significantly increased practice net without reducing the staff compensation. We have doubled practice incomes with high-density scheduling and staff leveraging methods. And we have given practice leaders more time with their families while increasing practice liquidity. These facts appear to reflect a basic restructure/redesign concern rather than a veterinary market concern.

We know that our profession often is fragmented—yet there are innovators like the Buffalo veterinary practices who cooperate monthly and bring outstanding continuing education to their community, or the Northwest Veterinary Managers Association who selflessly share trend information at their monthly meetings. We also know that most practices want to do better and will respond to positive guidance, rather than a list of negative "The Sky Is Falling" findings.

We hope this reference text provides the basis for many hours of practice discussion and debate, as well as new ideas and alternatives that previously seemed impossible. We have organized the most common practice management and leadership issues into general categories, and then included what we brain-stormed to be the most applicable alternatives for each. This arrangement allows the reader to have choices for positive and progressive action at his or her own level of commitment and capabilities. We wish for the reader to see that the "one best solution" of the past is not the best solution for the future. Most of all, it is our hope that the readers of this Secrets reference see the secrets of this profession as being founded in people, communication, and change, and see themselves as change agents for improving this profession we love and cherish.

1. STARTING YOUR PRACTICE

YOUR NEW CLINIC

1. Is there a simple business start-up checklist?

Starting a business is never simple, but the list below is meant to remind you of the tasks you may have to perform. Not every practice will require each step. For instance, you may decide not to register your trademark with state or federal officials, or you may not have to publish a notice of intent to do business. Since laws vary by state and community, especially for licenses and taxes, *be sure to check with local authorities* to determine if there are any additional legal steps you need to take (most have small business checklists).

• First, define what you will offer the community. This is called strategic positioning.
  • Determine who will buy services and how often. This is called setting goals.
  • Are you willing to do what it takes to operate during the hours the community needs?
  • Seek local advice from the Service Corps of Retired Executives or Americans Communicating Electronically (contact the Small Business Administration).
  • Know what it will cost to produce, advertise, sell, and deliver your services.
  • Assemble copies of the laws with which you will have to comply.
  • Define the line items so that you can make a profit on each.
  • Know how long it will take to make a profit as a business.
  • Write a business plan and a marketing plan.
  • Choose a practice name (localities have a better draw than surnames).
  • Verify right to use the name.
  • Reserve corporate name if you will be incorporating.
  • Register or reserve state or federal trademark.
  • Register copyrights.
  • Check zoning laws.
  • Choose locations for the practice.
  • File partnership or corporate papers.
  • Register practice name, and get a local business certificate.
  • Get any required business licenses or permits.

9

- Order any required notices (advertisements you have to place) of your intent to do business in the community.
- Have business phone lines installed (incoming, credit card, fax, and e-mail).
- Check into practice and personal insurance needs.
- Find out about health insurance for staff and yourself.
- Apply for sales tax number.
- Get tax information, such as recordkeeping requirements, information on withholding taxes if you will have employees, information on hiring independent contractors, facts about estimating taxes, and forms of organization.
- Call U.S. Department of Labor to determine applicable labor laws.
- Apply for employee identification number.
- Find out about workers' compensation.
- Open business bank account(s)—negotiate for sweeps and credit card rates.
- Have business cards and stationery printed.
- Purchase equipment and supplies.
- Order inventory, signage, and fixtures.
- Have practice literature prepared.
- Get adequate business insurance, liability insurance, and disability insurance.
- Send out publicity releases.
- Place only the advertising that will benefit your practice immediately.
- Call everyone you know and let them know you are in practice.
- Brainstorm other needs with your banker, accountant, lawyer, and consultant.

2. Where do I start?

The basis of any new endeavor is the basis of the business, and in veterinary medicine, that means centering on **healthcare programs**. New graduates have a tertiary care focus (required to pass boards), but the average practitioner has a client-centered focus. This focus in one of a patient advocate offering wellness programs and, occasionally, addressing sickness and/or injury. The "bread and butter" of most veterinary medical practices lies in the programs offered.

Veterinary healthcare programs are centered on the **core values** of the primary provider. In start-up practices, this is usually a "no-brainer" since there is no other staff. As a practice grows, however, the need to quantify and share the core values grows, but this communication seldom happens in an overt, premeditated manner.

3. What should my basic core values be?

No one can give you this answer. It is totally personal. However, consider the following examples:

• Over 30 years ago, Ray Kroc said you could train teenagers and, more importantly, form a successful workforce with them. He started with four core values, represented by Q-V-S-C: **quality, value, service,** and **cleanliness**. The job descriptions had four parts: Q-V-S-C. The operating procedures had four parts: Q-V-S-C. The merit pay increases came based on four parts: Q-V-S-C. McDonald's restaurants around the world were built on those simple value factors.

• In some progressive human healthcare facilities, "We CARE" represents the core values for the staff and providers: We = the accountable people in the delivery of quality healthcare and caring service; C = **Client** always comes first; A = **Action** is expected from every staff member; R = **Respect** for each individual, our staff as well as our clients; and E = **Excellence** in everything we do.

• We have offered PRIDE as a starting point for team discussion in some veterinary practices:

> P = **Patient first** (patient advocacy is our professional covenant)
> R = **Respect always** (respect, responsibility, recognition)
> I = **Innovation and ideas** (continuous quality improvement)
> D = **Dedication** (this profession is a calling, and clients demand it)
> E = **Excellence** (it is a "go–no go" standard in healthcare; expectations must be exceeded at all times!)

4. Why are core values so important?

Core values provide the yardstick for assessing the **mission focus** on every program a practice pursues. Mission focus is the application of core values to the standards of excellence required in veterinary healthcare delivery. The following sample mission statement demonstrates how core values augment a mission:

> *Provide quality healthcare delivery, while ensuring proper remuneration to the providers and facility, while establishing a community market niche.*

But mission statements do not make the programs work; people make the programs work! People need security in what they pursue, and since core values are inviolate, they provide the structure for tough program decisions.

5. What are the most profitable programs for my new practice?

In an equine practice, the most profitable programs are wellness programs. In a production practice, profit lies in well animals. In a companion-animal practice, the most profitable programs ensure healthy and happy animals in a household environment. In boarding operations, such programs offer a home-like environment to keep the stewards of the animals satisfied.

6. Aside from profit, what should programs provide?

The key programs must provide a feeling of "great, gee whiz, cool, and groovy" to the veterinary healthcare practitioner, the client, and the staff. The practitioner should feel accomplishment; the client should be satisfied and have peace of mind; and the staff should be full of pride. This latter benefit will be perceived as quality by clients, and clients pay happily for perceived quality.

The idea is to encourage everyone to get excited, feel the passion, be proud!

LOCATION—LOCATION—LOCATION

7. Describe some key location concerns.

Zoning, including environmental restrictions. The Design Start Kit for Veterinary Hospitals, 3rd edition, by Catanzaro (available from AAHA) has a good set of questions and personality profiles for self-assessment.

Curb cut locations. Can clients easily access the parking lot from the street? Or is it too busy; there are no cross-overs; they can get in but not out? These details vary with traffic count (highway traffic density).

Client location. Check where the clients are coming from, the locations of single-unit living areas, and routes to the supermarket, drug store, child-care center, and dry cleaners. A location that is demographically suited for day care or a stand-alone drug store also is compatible with a veterinary practice. A customer's choice of these facilities usually is based on home-to-site access, not drive-by impulse as in fast food or gasoline purchases.

Signage. Your sign must be visible to the traffic, and must allow advanced awareness of your driveway. Community sign codes can confuse this issue. Note that a time and temperature sign gets daily attention for your facility.

8. What is a catchment area?

A catchment area is the geographic area from which 80% of your clients will come. For a new practice in a metroplex area, it is the area circumscribed by the surrounding practices.

A new practice in an established area must virtually "steal" clients, since everyone already has a practice they frequent. In a growing community, look for the new start of housing areas (in the U.S., where there are no restraining boundaries or geographic barriers, most communities grow to the North and West).

9. What are FTE doctor computations?

The full time equivalent (FTE) doctor rating has become far more critical with the number of part-time veterinarians available for hire. The FTE computation allows a practice 25 minutes away with four doctors and a similar quality to be adjusted to one FTE impact on the potential catchment area (0.25 draw × 4 FTE doctors = 1 FTE). This perspective allows the established practice owner to see his or her practice as a demand for veterinary services, rather than a demand for personal time.

10. List the features I should seek when selecting a new site.

- Traffic counts are misleading, since pet owners must return home to get their pets. Look at demographics that are similar to stand-alone drug stores and childcare centers, which have similar domicile-distance patronage patterns.
- In average communities, $50–60 million of community income per FTE doctor impacting the catchment area.
- In average communities, 4000–5000 population per FTE doctor impacting the catchment area.
- In average communities, 1500–2000 companion animals per FTE doctor impacting the catchment area.
- No other practices within a 15-minute drive (this is just a wild dream in most metroplex areas).
- A boundary on the catchment area that opens to a larger, diverse population—without a blocking practice, geographic barriers, or psychological barriers.

11. Is there a good "rule of thumb" to use for sizing up the potential of a practice area?

There are many different ways to do this, but one quick and easy method starts with deciding **(1)** how much money you want to make from your practice (see the size and impact figures in Question 10), and **(2)** how much you have to invest in the start-up. Next, obtain a population count for the area you intend to serve (usually available at the public library, city hall, a marketing research firm, or a reputable veterinary consulting firm).

- Estimate the number of households (HH) by dividing the population by two.
- Estimate the number of pet-owning HH by multiplying by 0.60.

- Estimate the total number of pets for these HH by multiplying by 1.5.
- Reduce the total number of pets you might expect to see by how many pets you estimate are already being cared for by other veterinarians in the area.
- Multiply the remaining number of pets by 1.5 to 4.5 veterinary visits per year (average number of times you expect to see client per year).
- Multiply this number by your average client transaction (ACT) to estimate your annual gross income.
- Subtract your estimated expenses and taxes from this number.
- Does the remaining number match or exceed the amount you needed to make? If not, are housing tracts going up that would increase the population and pet ownership of the area? Or is there something that you could change to increase revenue, like the amount of your ACT or the average number of times you see each pet in your office?

Note that the Chamber of Commerce may be able to provide some of the above data.

FINANCING YOUR DREAM

12. Where do I get the money to start my practice?

An investment by extended family, minor savings, or your own credit cards usually can finance a store-front companion animal veterinary practice (< $20,000 for an economical start).

An ambulatory, equine, or house-call veterinarian may invest in a vehicle and use a garage for inventory, until some savings can be amassed for a facility. Vehicle purchase does not fall within traditional facility lending ratios (home < 28% gross taxable income, and facility plus consumer debt < 36% gross taxable income).

All that is required is a leasehold allowance from the landlord, two consultation rooms, and a reception and waiting area between the consultation rooms and front door. Everything behind the consultation rooms can be finished later.

The initial procurement of drugs from a distributor usually can be put on delayed payment with no interest, so don't use your credit card for the initial inventory. You don't need the credit card interest building up!

13. What about money sources if I want to start with a free-standing facility?

In parts of this country, banks will competitively bid for the right to loan you money for a veterinary hospital. Lenders like the Money Store are actually soliciting veterinary borrowers, since veterinarians are such a good credit risk.

14. Describe other concerns in starting a free-standing facility.

Land must be found that is at the right place at the right time for new clients; you must be flexible. The land should be separately deeded and owned from the practice because it is likely to become a long-standing family asset, since most dirt never decreases in value.

The **building** will appear when you are willing to spend $150 per square foot for construction costs and for at least 2500 square feet. This size means having minimal runs in the kennel space, no boarding or grooming, and probably only three consultation rooms.

Equipment can be added slowly. Radiography, ECG, ultrasound, and other imaging services can be coordinated with a neighboring practice, as can surgery suite time. These two areas of most hospitals have significant "dark time."

15. Should I seek professional advice when financing my business?

Yes! Regardless of money source, always have your attorney and accountant look at the contract for balloon payment options, prepayment penalties, and the cost of loan interest and fees. It is amazing how many contracts are never negotiated . . . and yes, you even can negotiate with a bank.

LEASEHOLD VERSUS FREE-STANDING

16. Why are leaseholds usually store fronts?

The usual economical space available for a start-up veterinary practice is 1400–2000 square feet in a shopping center (a leasehold)—all the new veterinarian must do is build the interior to start his or her dream. Some have been built for as little as $50 per square foot, but most are closer to $100 a square foot due to plumbing and electrical requirements. Note that a landlord may or may not give a leasehold allowance, but it is *always* a negotiable item.

Some practitioners offer their practices for lease, but buying veterinarians typically shy away from this option due to the low cost of a leasehold site. Remember that by leasing a practice, you gain an immediate client base.

17. Why are free-standing facilities so sought after?

• A free-standing facility generally offers an equity position concurrent with building a practice.

• No landlord (except yourself) means never having to say "may I?" and allows a feeling of freedom, which is a reason many enter this profession.

• The external design of a free-standing facility (e.g., architecture, signage) can be structured to attract drive-by traffic.

- The zoning on a free-standing piece of property often allows special use that is more compatible with veterinary facilities, whether it be overnight animals or chemotherapy waste elimination.
- A free-standing facility allows landscaping to match the decor (this may be good or bad, depending on your green thumb).

18. Is a store front or stand-alone best?

The store-front clinical facility is a more economical alternative for start-ups, since there are no land or exterior structure purchases. Rent does not build equity, but leasehold improvements allow extra tax deductions.

A stand-alone hospital is a greater debt expense, but also a potential equity investment. It also provides a greater attraction to drive-by clients—about a 15–20% increase in traffic for the first year.

A pet-center complex combines the attributes of a stand-alone facility with the economies of scale of a store-front complex, but adds the challenge of managing boarding, bathing, boutique, and grooming operations.

While human healthcare has evolved the neighborhood "doc in the box" concept for ease of access, the density of veterinary practices does not afford that convenient image. The decision to start or buy a store-front practice must be based on the **economy of the decision**, not the image of the veterinary practice.

BUDGETING

19. What use is a budget in a veterinary practice?

The new practice must submit to a budget to any lending institution to illustrate a business awareness of income and expense. The traditional budget prepared by accountants is expense-based and shows the historical spending of the practice. The traditional accountant puts a disclaimer on the front of each financial statement (third or fourth paragraph) that says, in effect, "Do not trust anything we say; it is unsubstantiated." Since most practices get their expenses under control within two to three business cycles, the continuous reproduction of expense-based budgets becomes redundant and no longer meaningful.

We recommend an aggressive, program-based budget, since programs change on a regular basis. The relationship between income and expense by line item must be appreciated to capture net income.

20. How can I use a program-based budget in practice?

A program is a commitment to some aspect of income production, such as equine dentistry, surgery, nutrition, holistic medicine, vaccinations, geriatrics, puppy/kitten wellness protection, dental prophylactic procedures, pain management, pre-anesthetic laboratory screening, or radiology. A host of other ideas are emerging in this profession. Annual budget planning involves serial application of core values to veterinary healthcare programs to produce an estimate of administration frequency. When coupled with realistic pricing, the net per procedure can be estimated and entered into the practice's program-based budget.

A program-based budget allows actual healthcare delivery to be compared to the estimated levels of program commitment. Individual adjustments can be made to improve the success rate of the program delivery.

The veterinary program-based budget is a form of written conscience for planning self-assessment of new program delivery. (See Chapter 4 of *Building The Successful Veterinary Practice: Programs & Procedures* [Volume 2] for operator-level details on program-based budgeting. This book is listed here in Appendix D.)

21. What should I look for in my accountant's reports?

Balance sheets are critical, as are income statements (profit and loss [P&L] reports). A statement of cash position is important if the accountant is providing an accrual report. Most accountants do not detail income centers (they are not needed by the IRS), and the most current accounting services convert the practice's cash basis accounting to accrual (another response to the IRS, as promoted by the AVMA), so accountant reports are not easily converted.

Many accountants alphabetize the expenses on the P&L, but cannot spell "accounting" (since if they could, it would appear as the first line item). They place accounting fees under "Legal," "Professional Fees," or other confusing categories. As you build your fiscal reporting system, require the accountant to use the categories as described by the practice (unless *they* are paying *you* to use their chart of accounts).

22. Do you have any tips for working with an accountant?

Accountants know their clients read from top to bottom and put more weight on the first things they read, so this tells savvy practitioners what to *require* in their tasking letter to their accountant: follow the sequence of the AAHA Chart of Accounts for the balance sheet and P&L expenses! An expanded and improved AAHA Chart of Accounts version is published in the appendices of *Building The Successful Veterinary Practice: Programs & Procedures* (Volume 2).

Ideally, practices should be using software called QuickBooks by Intuit (over 10 million users can't be wrong), or a similar "client-friendly" check-writing system so they can produce their own monthly P&L and balance sheet—in real time, on a cash basis. Then the accountant need only take the practice-developed monthly reports and generate a single quarterly report, converting to accrual for estimating taxes.

23. Who should be on my business team?

The practice accountant should be a **business tax accountant** and should stay aware of rulings affecting professional corporations (especially veterinarians).

The practice bank should have assigned a **personal business banker** who will discuss contingency lines of credit, equipment lines of credit, refinancing options for expensive leases, money market sweep accounts for deposits, and economical credit card services.

There needs to be a skilled **corporate attorney**, one who understands veterinary medical operations and legal considerations for professional groups.

The use of a veterinary-exclusive, multi-consultant, diversified, ethical **consulting firm** to coordinate the other professionals on the business team, as well as advise on operational issues, program-based budgeting process, and staff training programs, is highly recommended for most veterinary practices.

At the web site www.v-p-c.com, there is a list of suggested parameters for selecting a practice consultant, as well as criteria of ethical consulting. These lists were developed a few years ago by the Veterinary Consultant Network, a loose affiliation of over 45 nationally recognized veterinary-exclusive consultants, as a service to the veterinary profession.

24. How do I keep telephone bills down?

Think about how your company telephones will be used. According to the results of a study of messaging systems conducted by Gallup/Pitney Bowes, a whopping 41% of the average annual phone bill at Fortune 500 companies is attributable to fax calls.
- 60% of daily fax users are sending more faxes this year than last and claim it is more reliable and generates faster response than e-mail, voice mail, and overnight courier.
- Many companies are still using older, slower, stand-alone faxes; 60% of telecommunications managers believe that faster fax machines could substantially reduce their phone bills.

If you or your staff will use fax transmissions extensively, and if you have an older fax, upgrading to a faster model could help you cut your phone bill. If you plan on using a model with thermal paper and then photocopying the faxes you receive to make more permanent copies, consider switching to a plain paper fax—it could further reduce your costs.

For on-the-road long distance, take a pre-paid calling card along. It will save you money over the high surcharges hotels add to phone calls dialed directly from your room, and usually is cheaper than a phone company calling card, too.

COMPUTERIZATION

25. How can I pick the right computer system for my practice?

Most standard veterinary computer systems of the past two decades have been electronic cash registers hooked to word processors with a mail-merge feature. This is rapidly changing, and touch screens, the ability to add pictures to medical records, and integrated appointment logs all are great and available. The processors are getting faster, and laser and ink-jet printers now replace dot-matrix printers in almost all applications because they are quieter, faster, and cheaper.

During the initial system screening, count how many times the vendor tells you something to the effect, ". . . you will only need to modify your practice style a little. . ." While some practice documentation methods may need to be modified, invite back only those who are willing to *modify their system rather than your practice philosophy.*

The system must be selected on predetermined practice needs. The decision should depend on the staff's computer literacy, the vendor service support of the locality, and the philosophy of the practice—not the salesman's opinion. Keep control of the selection process, and computerization will not hurt . . . honest!

Tips For Selecting a Computer System

- The longer a computer product has been on the market, the greater the chance for increased savings.
- Technological upgrades sometimes are missing from the older systems. Don't discount vendors that you've never heard of in favor of a brand name. Remember that even Intel, Microsoft, and America Online were "newbies" once!
- Arrange for a private demonstration. Let the vendor know that this will be the first part of a two-step process—*if* they make the final cut, you will ask them back to demonstrate their system again (indicates you're not going to be pressured into signing a contract that day).
- Tell the vendor to show you how their system accomplishes tasks on your list; don't accept a prepared "demo" outlining features.

Table continued on next page.

Tips For Selecting a Computer System (Continued)

- Have each person on your team rate (1-weak to 5-great) each system according to ease of doing tasks and personal impression of output. Add up the numbers for each system and compare.
- Eliminate any system that can't do a critical task.

26. How do I narrow the field to a single computer?

There are differences in the "feel" between programs, but not many in the actual capabilities (e.g., they all do invoicing, reminders, and prescription labels, but some require many screens to get it done, or cannot reverse screens and require you to go through the whole process before correcting an entry error).

After the initial selection of qualified applicants, **re-evaluate** the top three contenders. You may be confused with the minute details after looking at so many choices, and your criteria list may need to be rewritten before this final selection phase.

There should be some onsite **personnel training** time included in each purchase. Vendors typically offer some form of basic training system as part of the total package, with the intent of selling you more, but the time onsite (initial and followup) is the most negotiable aspect of the contract.

Some vendors offer offsite support at a supplemental fee to the maintenance fee. Be sure to compute all the out-year costs, supplemental training costs for new staff, and system upgrade costs when comparing systems.

27. Where should I buy the computer system hardware?

When speaking of Windows-based software and the actual computer, make sure you understand the vendor's position on hardware. Some veterinary computer software companies sell systems to a practice without supplying the associated hardware components. Some won't supply the hardware no matter how much you beg!

Advantage to having the software company supply the hardware: it's easier to deal with the inevitable problems that arise because one company is responsible for everything.

Disadvantages: possible higher-than-market prices for components, and return of device for servicing. Note that you can require the software vendor to supply a technical sheet showing all the hardware requirements, as a basis for comparison of costs.

Obtaining the hardware from a local computer supplier typically is the least expensive alternative, and having a person available for servicing is a definite plus, but it has its downside as well. When something goes wrong, it's often an exercise in frustration dealing with two technical support departments—the hardware people say it's a software problem, and the software people say it's a hardware problem.

28. What training should I expect from the vendor?

If you or a staff member is computer-savvy, the Windows-based systems may require minimal instruction from the vendor. You may be able to focus on **tailoring the system** to be practice specific.

If you have absolutely no interest in becoming a "techno geek" yourself, and you don't have one on staff, instruction on basic computer operation will be necessary. Be sure to negotiate the best deal you can on the level of training you receive.

No matter what your skill level on the computer, when the vendor's trainer is onsite, be sure to capture as much knowledge as possible. Don't rely on any training schedule of theirs; have your list of tasks available (the one you made during the evaluations), and make it the training agenda once the system is up and running.

Expect a clear and refined **user's manual**—it may be on paper, in the software, or on the Internet. Be sure the manual matches the system generation you are buying (some vendors are infamous for being behind in updating their software user's manual). If this valuable tool is missing, you will be at the mercy of the vendor's technical representative on the other end of the phone.

The absence of a good user's manual may indicate that the software is still in "alpha" or "beta" testing. If you're comfortable with considering yourself a test site, you should negotiate a greater reduction in price.

29. How is computer training of new employees handled?

Now is the time to consider future training needs. Unless you want to pay the vendor for additional onsite training every time you hire a new staff member, you'll have to do the subsequent training inhouse. Video training is the most effective and easily replicated form of computer training available, but few vendors have taken the time to make instructional videos for their systems. You'll have to do this yourself:

• Don't worry about the technical quality of the video (e.g., lighting, sound); focus on capturing the information that must be taught.

• Set up a video camera on a tripod near the computer so that it captures the keyboard and screen. Now every word that is spoken and every key that is touched is recorded for use later with new staff members.

• Make a copy of the tape and keep it in a safe place in case the original is damaged or lost.

• Now you can train a new employee without huge time commitments from the rest of the practice team!

30. What are critical hardware specifications for supporting veterinary software?

Look at the central processing unit (CPU) speed and available random-access memory (RAM): you cannot get enough of either, so upgrade and expansion is critical. The "mother board" is likely to have a speed upgrade in the near future, so know the upgrade costs of each element of your hardware.

31. Do you have any tips for saving money?

There is strength in bargaining; list prices are a starting point. In 1992, IBM, Apple, and others removed suggested resale value prices from their products (deregulated). The hardware market is now consumer-driven, and the technology changes so fast that "bigger and better" no longer creates demand.

If your practice is bargaining for multiple printers or multiple terminals, don't be afraid to argue for a lower price. There is a long tradition of haggling in the computer business, so *do not meekly accept the list price.* Conversely, if you are buying a single-user system, your bargaining strength is greatly reduced.

Factor in all costs. Does the system come with onsite service? If so, at what cost? Some mail-order vendors guarantee overnight replacement parts, and some in-city sources have to send the hardware out of state for repairs; the difference can be significant. How are problems diagnosed? Do you need a dedicated modem or is it done over the phone? (You want to avoid 2 A.M. emergency calls.) Who disassembles and assembles the system? Any maintenance agreement must address downtime as well as replacement costs; assess the direct and indirect expense of both.

32. Is leasing a good idea?

Some companies suggest that a lease is the only way to procure rapidly changing technology. From an objective, fiscal point of view, leasing is a bum deal: the cost is greater than the purchase price, and the service is about equal to outright ownership programs. Most leases are 36-month, expiring long before the computer system becomes obsolete. The ability to upgrade varies with the lease, as do the maintenance responsibilities. With the ever-changing tax laws, tax advantages of purchase versus lease can change often, so check with your accountant before making this decision.

33. What should I know about negotiating the computer contract?

No sophisticated purchaser signs a standard computer contractual agreement without modification.

—L. Sherwin, J.D. Memel

One of the first principles to accept is that the negotiation process itself has value, as it exposes the vendor's willingness and capabilities to meet your specific practice needs. During negotiation, problem solving occurs in a noncrisis setting, and the practice-vendor relationship gains confidence and security.

The second principle to accept: most vendor computer contracts are relatively short, standard documents that fail to adequately cover the details of the transaction. Presented details often are slanted toward the vendor and offer very limited protection to the purchaser. These standard contracts offered to veterinary medical practices seldom reiterate the claims made in the promotional literature or by the vendor's representative.

Tips For Drawing Up the Contract

- Keep good notes, and read the whole contract. Amend it by adding the promotional literature, vendor claims, and sales quotes as contractual guarantees (addendums).

- Contracts *can* be changed, despite the vendor's statements to the contrary. Equally false is the notion that only minor changes can be inserted (ask your attorney). Beware if the sales representative "promises" to cover for the "company's shortfall" in the contract: If it isn't committed in writing and attached to the contract as an official enclosure, it has no value!

- Most lawyers agree that the party who initially drafts the agreement has the advantage. Consider having your attorney draft a completely new contract. He or she can follow the vendor's format, and even incorporate some of the same terminology. Starting fresh gives the purchase clarity; addenda, inserts, and added clauses generally are too brief to allow a clear expression of the total intent of the change. Let the vendor work from and make changes to *your* document.

- The party seeking to make changes in someone else's document always is at a psychological disadvantage. Many traditional computer vendors are fond of accusing veterinarians, ". . . those changes are nitpicky" or ". . . unreasonable." Work toward receiving this compliment, because if they don't say it, you haven't pushed them far enough!

34. What are some key computer contract issues?

Hold the vendor responsible for claims made. All of the promotional literature and brochures that show specifications and benefits should be incorporated into the contract. Only then can you hold the vendor responsible if the products do not perform.

Ensure performance. Use terms that define the product performance. Speed, capacity, vendor's obligations, and updates to achieve performance (modifications, enhancements, refinements, and improvements always should be no cost provisions of purchase) should be provided on each element of the system to ensure that there is a clear warranty and maintenance commitment concurrent with the contract acceptance date (rather than the delivery date).

Put your purchase to work. Installation and training often are vague or unspecified in vendor contracts. Clear responsibilities and timetables must be set out. Pinpoint who will support your system, and maintain your right to a replacement person if you are dissatisfied. You can impose penalties on the vendor for failure of performance, so include a right of extrication. Regular status review meetings are not unrealistic terms for purchase, nor are 90-day and 6-month training refresher and update visitations.

Achieve satisfaction. An acceptance procedure should be part of the contract. It should be your right to run acceptance tests on your premises; define both the vendor's role and your role in the process; determine a timetable; and specify what happens if the product fails to perform. Test criteria can be incorporated into the agreement as an exhibit. The practice's payment periods should never start until *after* these test phases are successfully completed.

Arrange a favorable payment schedule. Although the vendor wants everything up front, seek to minimize any deposit and defer payment as long as possible to ensure satisfaction with the vendor's performance. Payment milestones, i.e., certain system events that will trigger a payment due date, should be clearly stated in the agreement and tied to the vendor's performance obligations.

Define warranty scope and duration. It is imperative that you clearly define the warranty scope and duration for *every element* of the system. Vendors often try to convince you that there is only a single "standard" clause, but this is far from accurate! Some subcategories to negotiate:

    a. Ensure *compatibility* with existing or currently purchased hardware and software.

    b. Specify *speed* for the tasks intended as performance specifications for the various configurations discussed or claimed by the vendor, regardless of whether initially purchased or installed.

    c. Require *service response* provisions, including what hours the vendor will be available and how fast they will respond, onsite vs. by telephone, and when replacement systems will be required. Provisions for escalating the problem up the vendor's executive ladder should be in the agreement, as well as the qualifications of the service personnel.

d. Allow for the *customization* of software after it has been used for a period of time, to make it more adequately meet your practice needs. These changes should not impact the warranty.
e. Release of *source codes* (programming details) is a must. This allows protection of the purchaser in cases where the vendor decides to cease support or update functions, for economic or other reasons.

Check the maintenance agreement. Again, never accept the standard clause. Some vendors offer free maintenance for a period after the warranty term, and it may be possible to negotiate a cap for annual maintenance fee increases.

Check plans for manufacturer's updating of the software. This needs to be done in a timely manner during the warranty. Maintenance periods must be specified to meet state and federal laws and regulations that impact the software program. Obtain the counsel of a competent attorney to better understand your rights.

35. How critical is the Windows operating platform?

The new diagnostic instruments as well as graphic systems are compatible with the Windows *and* Apple platforms (although there are far fewer Apple vendors in our profession, which should automatically tell you something). Thus, easy integration of multiple systems is possible. Changes in operational systems (e.g., Unix, Zenix, Aix) generally are included in software vendor upgrades.

Both the Windows and Apple platforms make Internet access far easier. Any practice not on the Internet will be left behind!

36. List some critical points for concern regarding operation of veterinary software.

- Count the times any vendor says, "You only have to change a little ..." during the discussions, since this indicates the gap between what you want and what they have to offer.
- Review the appointment log. See how easily the appointment times can be changed, within a column as well as between columns. Determine how a doctor can be scheduled into two rooms, out of sync, for high-density scheduling.
- Review how easy it is to change the narratives on the reminder cards, and how easily the merge is to change from postcards to letters to envelopes to e-mail.
- Look at the inventory management module for ease of changing dispensing fees, minimum charges, surcharges for controlled substances, seasonal reorder points, and vendor history evaluations.

- Review how easy it is to go back and make a change on a previous screen, and look at what the transaction count becomes when you store an inpatient record and reopen it again later—is it double-counting these records?
- See if transactions and procedures track cleanly, even on bundled items, so you can look at the dollars per procedure at a later time.

37. My veterinary software system does a great job at tracking my income, but how do I keep better track of my expenses?

Any commercial bookkeeping system is acceptable if the bookkeeper is properly trained on the program and he or she follows the guidelines for income center posting. Otherwise, the best bookkeeping program to get is the one that is easiest to learn and use.

38. What is the best accounting software?

QuickBooks is the most popular, but there are many others. The managerial accounting is different from tax accounting (done by the CPA). You need to do your own managerial accounting, as you write and categorize checks, to be compatible with the AAHA Chart of Accounts (see Question 22) and to make informed economic decisions for your practice.

The ability to print a P&L statement and a balance sheet at the end of each month (within 72 hours to compare with the veterinary software output of income and procedures) allows you to do program-based budgeting.

The secret is in the people, not the software. Allocating costs to expense centers that match the veterinary software income centers is simply good business, but it's seldom done by veterinary practice software. This discipline must be started early in the evolution of the practice.

39. If I use QuickBooks, can I fire my accountant?

No. They fulfill two different functions. **Management bookkeeping** is simply the input of data in a specific way so as to produce information (reports) that tell the leadership about performance of the key areas of the business. **Tax accounting** is the application of available laws to exclude as much income as possible from taxation.

The accountant is a vital part of the practice management team. However, you can decrease the cost of the accountant by performing some or all of the bookkeeping tasks in-house. That way you provide the accountant with useable information, and he or she doesn't have to spend time organizing tons of raw data to do the job.

40. Does our practice really need to use the Internet?

Yes. The Internet is fast becoming the communication medium of the age. The immediate availability of information anywhere in the world at any

time of day means that it is here to stay. Learn to use the resources of the Internet so that you can:
- continue learning through online courses, interact with other professionals, and search for answers to challenges of the practice
- communicate with and educate clients or prospective clients (a practice-building tool)

41. How will the Internet benefit the practice?

Internet Features Beneficial to a Veterinary Practice

E-mail—communicate with colleagues, vendors, and staff members within a practice (Intranet).
- Employee notices and reminders automated, customized, and trackable
- A permanent record of the staff member receiving it

Web page for education of clients—most significant business use of the Internet; also allows delivery of a controlled image of the business
- Making appointments on-line still a way off for most practices.
- Give "phone shoppers" the web site address for more information.
- Within a defined community, having a web site is emerging as the differentiation factor among practices!

Continuing education (CE)—best thing to come along for personal growth in years! Taking medical and management CE courses right over the computer now commonplace.

Veterinary Information Network (www.vin.com) and the **Veterinary Support Personnel Network** (www.vspn.org)—premier spots for veterinary professionals to learn and interact

Peer-to-peer message boards—one of fastest ways to get answers to difficult cases, from specialists and general practitioners all over the world. Often, answers available within hours. Try that with a referral!

Research—easy to stay abreast of current government requirements (used to involve either advice of someone who was supposedly knowledgeable, or trial and error)
- Almost all government agencies now publish their regulations on the Internet, along with guides and resources to help in compliance.
- Major resource: availability of Material Safety Data Sheets online. Means drastic reduction in phone calls and letters because you can print them in your office.

Ordering supplies—fast becoming a way of life; major retail chains already use web-based ordering for office and computer supplies.
- Most veterinary distributors have web sites available for product information
- Soon you'll be able to place an order, check on status, and review your account.

42. What is the downside to Internet access?

Of course, with each new opportunity comes abuses. The same is true for the Internet in many ways.

- The act of venturing out on the Internet or sharing e-mail with others opens up the company computer system to potential problems.
- Viruses and "hacking" are concerning, but there are easy ways to protect the company.
- "Firewalls" and virus scan programs are effective tools; when used properly they virtually eliminate risk.
- It's easy to spend hours online searching and exploring. That's a personal choice on one's own time, but at work there are limits.

43. What are some guidelines for employee "surfing"?

Every practice should have Internet access so that the entire staff can learn, but a specific **Internet use policy** should be in effect. Access for checking e-mail can be unlimited. However, you might prohibit searching for, viewing, downloading, or printing pornography and hate-related or otherwise objectionable material from the company's computers. Daily time limits on the number of duty hours that any one staff member can access the Internet are a good idea. Note that some practices require each staff member to monitor different professional bulletin boards for interesting messages and provide brief reports at staff meetings.

44. Why is online continuing education beneficial?

Many practices offer a CE allowance to the staff, but sometimes it's not enough to cover registration and expenses. Moreover, it's not always convenient to be away for a week. Since most states now accept formal online CE courses for credentialing credits, more and more staff members are finding this an alternative to the traditional lecture.

In some ways, online CE is even better—the lessons are more interactive and, since they usually are spread out over weeks instead of hours, the staff member actually learns more. In most classes, the student is required to prepare materials under the guidance of the instructor that benefit the practice, and there are tests and quizzes to ensure that the student is keeping up with the material. When was the last time you got that at a formal meeting?!

45. Do I need a web site for my hospital?

Web sites can be a lot of fun, but they also are a lot of work. Unlike a Yellow Pages ad, they need constant updating and maintenance because Internet surfers have certain expectations for a web page.

Web pages should be visually engaging. In most cases they should be linked with the community Chamber of Commerce web site, since most newcomers check here for reputable businesses. Web pages must be easy to navigate, so that the user can find what is wanted without wading through everything else. The Internet is a highly visual medium: pictures are essential! Make your practice's web page interactive, and change it frequently so that there is always something new to see.

Veterinarians usually do not sell products or schedule appointments through the Internet; thus, advertising in the Yellow Pages is a far better investment for most hospitals (see Chapter 7). Times are changing fast, and the Internet is something to consider now so that you will be in the position to upgrade as it becomes a better business tool for general practice.

46. When using Internet marketing, how do we show visitors the way back to our site?

If you are doing a good job of marketing your web site—getting it listed in search engines and linked to other sites, especially the community's Chamber of Commerce—new visitors will find your web site every day of the week. If you have good content, friendly pictures, and information on your site, visitors may print it out for future reference. But what happens when they pull that printout from their files a month or two later? Will they remember your website address? Don't count on it. Additionally, if they reached your site through a link from another web site, there's a chance that the originating site will prevent your address from being shown. Make sure visitors can find their way to you by including your address in text at the bottom of every web page.

Marketing tip: always include information for new residents, such as animal control numbers, community standards for rabies and leash laws, and names of kennels where they can keep their animals while moving in.

EQUIPMENT AND INVENTORY

47. Which equipment is critical for a new practice?

It depends on your business arrangement: purchase, lease, or cooperation with established facilities. Diagnostic equipment for a "gate-keeper" practice (one that refers most cases to specialists) is less than that for a full-scope general practice in rural America. But even metroplex practices that share capital equipment resources can turn a better net.

Much of the basic equipment is available, in used condition, from veterinary schools. The question to consider is what is *required* versus what is nice to have. If there is not a good local laboratory, then a dry chemistry machine is needed. If you can find an inexpensive second-hand machine, it can be an immediate help and can provide a trade-in value (we know of clients who bought second hand for < $250 and obtained $5000 trade-in value).

Generally, the most costly single piece of essential diagnostic equipment is a 300 mA X-ray machine plus automatic processor (automatic processor generally provides 35% more income than hand-tank developing practices). Options are: community affiliation with established practices, lesser mA machines, reconditioned second-hand machines, and human healthcare cast-offs. Remember, few clients understand the difference between offsite and onsite services, and they won't care unless you make an issue of the matter. Many gate-keeper practices sell the advantage of limited services as a cost savings for clients (outpatient companion animal facilities can generate twice the net of a full-service veterinary facility).

SAFETY ALWAYS!

48. How do I keep up with all of the OSHA requirements?

First, realize that the safety of your staff and clients is paramount. Then establish the goal of a safe facility, inside and out, for clients, patients, and staff. *This is not a hassle; it is caring!*

Second, use the Internet for the most current information, but ensure you are dealing with veterinary-specific and knowledgeable people (e.g., Veterinary Information Network, Network of Animal Health [NOAH], and other reputable groups).

Third, procure the basic OSHA self-assessment package, from sources like AAHA or on the Internet at www.v-p-c.com for the veterinary-specific packages.

49. Where can I get the key elements for a veterinary safety program?

The Right to Know Program, Chemical Hazard Communication Program, and Radiation Safety Program all offer industry support, such as vendor Material Safety Data Sheet booklets, state/province radiation inspection programs, and similar regulatory efforts. Zoonotic diseases, mechanical injury, and women in the workplace often require veterinary-specific assistance to tailor programs to the practice. Disability concerns, like pregnancy or broken bones, require a physician's involvement so that employee limitations can be conveyed to the employer (practice owner).

Every practice should obtain *Veterinary Safety and Health Digest*, which provides basic, bimonthly updates (www.v-p-c.com/Phil/OSHA/links.htm). This publication usually deals with just one or two topics per issue, so the practice has ongoing reminders about safety upgrades.

EARLY STAFFING

50. Who are the first employees I should seek?
• A veterinarian who believes in quality healthcare and staff leadership, and who has a strong, client-centered, patient-advocacy approach in every consultation
• A client-centered veterinary technician (might even be called a "veterinary nurse" if the doctor is *really* client-centered)
• A caring receptionist (maybe your favorite host or hostess from a local restaurant). Fill this slot when you achieve your first $1000 day.

51. What is a fair way to establish compensation rates for staff?
Communities vary, but there are a few known starting points based on the employment market. The **equivalent method** allows comparables that are community specific. The "hiring wage" for untrained people should be slightly above the fast-food worker wage, with a raise when they start working solo (about 30 days into training/orientation), and a second increase at the end of the 90-day introductory period (based on competency, practice contributions, and team fit). The goal at the first anniversary is for the wage to be slightly above the assistant manager's wage at the local midscale department store.

The total **W-2 compensation package** (clinical wage for all doctors, administrative wages, and staff wages) for a companion-animal practice should not exceed 43% of gross any quarter. Specialty practices can increase that percentage by up to 5% due to the higher net within the individual invoice. Mixed-animal practices have such a variably low net on production animal drugs, that a lower percentage of gross often is required.

The receptionist, nurse technician, and animal caretaker percentages vary greatly by the practice philosophy and scope of services, but boarding and grooming operations must be separated from the practice budget before computing staff compensation targets.

Typically, the balance between the staff wage and the doctor's clinical compensation starts staff light (~18–19% staff and ~22–23% doctor). As the staff accepts more client outreach accountability, the balance shifts to the staff because they become veterinary extenders (~21–22% staff and ~19–20% doctor).

Note that pay periods should be twice a month to allow the best budget comparisons.

52. What is an acceptable doctor's wage?

In a mature companion-animal practice, you can hire as many doctors as the practice can hold if the W-2 compensation package is held to 20% and the benefits are less than 4%. The remaining 76% will support the well-managed practice overhead and leave an appropriate return on investment (excess net) for the practice owner.

Starting doctor (new graduate) wages vary by area and are increasing every year. About $40,000 (± 10%) the first year, during training and development of wellness healthcare delivery skills (primary care), is not unrealistic. Subsequent annual compensation may be 19–20% of the doctor's personal production during the last 6 months of the first employment year, times two—especially for a doctor who is training staff while delivering quality healthcare.

$$(.19 \times \text{production @ 6 months}) \times 2 = \text{salary}$$

In ensuing years, doctors should receive 19–20% of their previous year's personal production as base salary, with an increase of 0.5% each year they exceed their previous year's production by 10% or when they accept a management function that takes them off-line from production.

Ambulatory veterinarians, without haul-in facility capability, can receive as high as 40% compensation if there is no benefit package. Specialty practices can give associate board-certified specialists 30% (as low as 25% for board-qualified but not certified, and as high as 35% for board-certified specialists on the track to ownership).

53. How do I find good people to hire?

Hiring and firing are not secret management methods: **retention and training** are what make a successful veterinary healthcare team! The job description(s) outlines the practice's commitment to train the candidate to the appropriate skills and knowledge level during the 90-day orientation (and probation) period.

A practice's hiring team should include a trainer from each zone of the facility. The candidate has 90 days to demonstrate fit (harmony) and skills (competencies). These two characteristics must be present in anyone admitted to the practice's healthcare team.

Receptionists are responsible for client relations first and computer operations second. Notice people in client-contact positions (e.g., food service, department stores), and when someone impresses you, give them a business card and say, "If you ever want to get out of the food service business, give me a call. I can use someone with your attitude and people skills in our hospital's client relations program."

If you have accepted this method—hiring for attitude; training to provide skills and knowledge; and "growing" your own staff—use the Internet to help you out (e.g., online AVMA credentialed veterinary technician programs, AVMA study interactive staff development texts, AAHA training videotapes, CD-ROM learning sessions, and a host of other resources).

54. What is the best way to attract good employees?

Start by creating a clear concept of the kind of practice culture you want. What do you value: high quality medicine? workplace harmony? high profitability? client goodwill? challenging medicine? the regard of your peers? working the least amount of time possible? You can then hire prospective employees that fit your culture, and they will know why they're there and what they're supposed to do.

Additionally, here are some benefits that will help you make your practice attractive:
- Competitive pay (within community, not just within profession)
- Continuing education and/or degree completion (distance learning)
- Flexible scheduling
- Paid vacation time and sick leave (personal days)
- A 401k or other investment retirement plan
- Health benefits

55. How do I know when to fire someone?

Terms of employment must be clear from the first day. They should be developed around the core values of the practice so that everyone knows exactly what is expected. During the first 90 days, the candidate must learn to accept and embrace these core values, or they should be released from their temporary employment status (at will) before they contaminate the team.

"De-hire" employees when they have lost team fit or personal competency, or when they are no longer willing to support the practice's healthcare delivery programs. As a practice evolves to better meet the needs of the community, people who fight for the past (anti-change) are doomed to relive it, so they should be released to seek their own horizons.

A practice must pursue continuous quality improvement to survive. Each staff member must be willing to make changes in his or her own sphere of influence to improve tomorrow, next week, and next month. Let your people know that they should expect de-hiring if they fail to embrace change.

56. Firing is difficult. Is there an easy way?

Firing is difficult because most doctors have clear-cut expectations for job performance, but are still used to the school system for grading performance: A = excellent, B = above average, C = average, D = below average, F = unacceptable. This grading system allows many gray areas. Compromising between these two ideals—the "black and white" method and the "gray areas" method—is difficult. Most doctors question where to draw the line, and this uncertainty causes unclear measurements of performance. Without clear standards, the decision to "de-hire" is very difficult.

First, ensure that the core values are clear to each and every person on the team. Second, ensure each variant from the standard is addressed immediately with training, counseling, and one-on-one statements of expected behavior in the future.

When new endeavors are initiated, evaluate training by observing individuals during practical application. Recognize success with public celebration (counsel in private). When an employee diverts from the practice direction or standards of excellence, de-hiring may be needed. Consider that you simply are allowing the individual the opportunity to seek another work environment that better suits his or her skills and attitude. The employee is not a bad person; he or she just did not grow with the practice's direction.

57. We have been growing so fast that the staff is leaving due to the pressures. How do we keep good people?

Fast growth is always stressful, so keep it light; make humor and laughter an integral part of the practice culture.

In a fast-paced practice, decisions often are stove-piped. Get everyone involved in the client-centered service mission and thinking like patient advocates, and ask leading questions of the team *before* making a policy decision or change in the established processes.

When business is brisk, the clients' needs often become secondary to healthcare delivery. These entities are codependent, so have the staff participate in some form of client survey and satisfaction inquiry, including making remedial responses to the findings.

Increased demands can be dehumanizing. Patients become syndromes; clients become numbers; and caring departs the practice's delivery process. Change the environment by changing labels: receptionists to "client relations specialists," technicians to "outpatient nurses," and animals to "patients in need." Also, have *the team* address how to improve the situation, and empower them to react and respond.

THE FRONT DOOR MUST SWING

58. Clients come in different shapes and sizes . . . what are they?

The **A client** visits the veterinarian multiple times a year and does whatever the doctor says is needed, when it is needed, with little thought about cost.

The **B client** visits the veterinarian multiple times a year and eventually does most of the things the doctor says are needed, with some concern about costs when they exceed the family budget threshold (about $500 per episode for 50% of pet owners).

The **C client** visits the veterinarian once a year, listens to what the doctor says is needed, and eventually makes a decision about the needs (usually after 5 or more exposures). The C client has strong concerns about veterinary costs as they relate to the family's discretionary income.

The **D client** visits the veterinarian irregularly, generally when healthcare or legal needs demand the action.

59. Can we attract new clients with coupons and free services?

Yes. However, a 20% discount requires a 500% increase in business in most practices just to break even . . . and this requires a great team to achieve!

The better-paying clients (categories A and B) do not follow coupons and free services unless a practice breaks a bond with them—we see this with the large pet supply retailers who offer veterinary services. The C and D clients follow the coupons and bargains, but they seldom visit their veterinarian 3 to 6 times a year like an A or B client.

Some metroplex families select two veterinary facilities—one quality practice that they trust for medicine and surgery, and one economical, fast-in and fast-out clinic for wellness services. A quality practice can offer both, with some planning!

60. How many transactions should I be doing as a first-year practice?

As many as you can. In the first year you will not exceed your capacity, only your sanity. The initial clients in a new practice include many animal owners who are "bad credit" at other practices. Asking about a client's previous veterinarian is an ethical method of determining where you want to fit in the professional community.

If you are following the fee schedules established by the pet health insurance industry, you should have $1000 day by the end of the first month, and drive at least $150,000 in the first year of a companion animal practice.

MARKETING OR CLIENT EDUCATION?

61. How do we get our first clients?

Most times your **sign** will be the first inducement for clients to enter your facility. Keep it simple. Remember that they have less than 5 seconds to read it as they drive by. The words Animal Hospital, Veterinary Clinic, or a similar mixture should stand out, and maybe a phone number if you are not in the yellow pages yet.

The **Yellow Pages** are important when clients are new to the area and looking for a veterinarian close to their home. A Yellow Pages ad does very little in an established community where word-of-mouth referral is the most significant promotional tool.

While surveys show that 60% of all new clients select their veterinarian based on location, many actually make the selection based on the **recommendations** of others (including pet stores, humane societies, and other animal adoption locations). Therefore, ensure that there is good will between you and the community. Start word-of-mouth promotion by speaking on a current hot topic at local homeowner groups, country clubs, civic organizations, schools, and similar high-profile organizations. You'll have the time to do this because you won't have clients keeping you busy.

Ask the local **newspaper** to run an article on you and your practice as a new business entering town. Have a "hook" that will excite them, either in diagnostic services (e.g., computerized imaging, automated radiology, allergy testing, surgical monitors) or in your facility design (e.g., cat condos, kitty gazebo in waiting area, special runs).

62. How can we target one preferred segment of the pet-owning population?

About 60% of clients choose their veterinarian from the selection available within a 15-minute drive from their home. In rural communities, this distance is extended and depends on the shopping habits of the community. About the same number also ask a neighbor or pet store about the quality of local veterinarians when making their choice. In mixed species practices, word-of-mouth is more significant than location, especially in production animal environments where pennies per hundred weight can make a profit difference.

Practices that join the Chamber of Commerce and have a page on the Chamber's website (or on other community-based websites) get some traffic due to "first known name" recognition factors. A few clients are referred from AAHA hospital to AAHA hospital. National awareness of the American Animal Hospital Association certification process is still minimal in most areas.

Note that a client who comes by word of mouth typically forgives a bad first impression, whereas coupon and discount clients react negatively and may start a word-of-mouth program giving you a bad reputation. A poor community reputation can take as long as 10 years to reverse, so client bonding is critical during the first visit.

63. What is the best method to increase our access to new clients?

Clients are community and practice specific, so there is no single best method. Retention and nurturing of existing clients feeds the word-of-mouth reputation, which is the strongest new-client program available.

Price-centered practices, like "shoot and scoot" vaccination clinics and "pay and spay" programs, deal strictly in volume, so the widest exposure possible is essential. Consider radio ads played during rush-hour traffic.

A **recovered client program** is a new twist, because it brings back the clients who selected the practice, but then did not return. At just one recovered client a day, 6 days a week, 50 weeks a year, with 1.5 pets per household and 4 visits per pet per year, annual net income can increase well over $100,000 without changing anything else in the practice.

64. What are the minimum essential services to offer in a new practice?

There is no menu of services for new practices and mate practices (i.e., satellite second practice with same owner). If you are going to bond with clients, start with a solid set of core values based on sound medical and surgical beliefs. Offer the best veterinary care by clearly stating needs, then be quiet until the client speaks. If you must speak after stating a need (yours or an animal's), only ask, "Is this the level of care you want for Spike today?"; then fall silent again.

Minimum essential services should include many "two-yes" options, such as: a titer screen and a vaccination, two-lead cardiac screen as well as a full seven-lead method, two types of electronic monitoring in surgery, two levels of preanesthetic screening, and/or two levels of pain management. Clients who are given two-yes choices at a new practice select appropriate care more than 75% of the time (in mature practices, this two-yes method moves positive responses to more than 95% of the time). When given a yes-no choice, 50% acceptance is a good rate.

Additionally, the minimum essential is a scope of services and products that is appropriate for you. An outpatient practice doesn't offer many inpatient services, and a specialty practice doesn't offer outpatient wellness care if they want to keep referrals coming from other veterinarians. Look in the mirror and determine what quality healthcare means to you, clearly state that belief to your staff, and then tell everyone in the practice how that belief is to be delivered to clients on the phone and in person. Narratives (scripts) must be solid in concept and believed by the speaker to sound authentic. Never let your phone or client narratives be just a set of words!

65. How can we make reminder cards more effective?

First, quit sending the code letters that come preprogrammed by some computer geek at the software company—what client really knows what FVRCP means?

It takes five or more exposures to get a "yes" when a client knows they need a service and over a dozen when they don't realize the importance. The reminder card is a call to action *following* these and other awareness exposures (e.g., newsletters, health alerts, consultation exposures).

A tag-line request added as a P.S. (postscript) will get as many responses as the basic message, since most people read P.S. messages first. They can double the potential response for a single mailing.

Reminders for dental services, geriatrics, exotics, internal parasite screens, external parasite screens, behavior management, nutritional programs, and related wellness care most often arrive as a "bolt from the blue," without preceding awareness or personal followup. Poor results are the result of single-shot reminder programs!

In today's market, an **annual life-cycle consultation** should replace the annual vaccines if a practice wants their clients to get into the proper habit of wellness visitation.

66. How do I build referrals to my general practice?

Find out where your new clients are coming from. If you are not collecting and tracking this information monthly, start now.

Ask each new client why they chose your practice. Was it your sign? Yellow Pages ad? Web site? Did another client refer them, and if so, who?

To reinforce word-of-mouth referrals, make sure that you:
- Thank whomever referred the client to you (by letter, phone, or in person the next time they come into the office).
- Track the number of referrals, and report it each month at your staff meeting to reinforce the importance of referrals to your staff. Talk about ways to increase the number of referrals.
- Display a tasteful sign in your reception area inviting clients to refer their friends and neighbors.
- Spoil your current clients to keep them high on you. Make a fuss over their pets and be pleasant and attentive to their needs.

67. List additional marketing ideas I can use to build my practice.

Participate in community pet-related causes, such as spay and neuter programs, pet adoption days, and pet walks, to gain favorable exposure for your practice. Make sure that the event planners publicize your participation and that you promote the event in your office.

Teach your staff how to "sell" on the phone. For instance, do they always invite the caller to come in, rather than just give out fee information to price shoppers? Or do they tell a client to wait for the doctor to call them back? Booking even two extra appointments a day easily adds over $2,500 a month to your gross, while improving the pet care of your patients.

68. What do I do when the guy down the road starts to bad mouth our work?

• **Keep a civil tongue** while taking defensive action. Speak no evil!

• **Spread the word.** Let all the staff and clients know up front that you will never engage in this type of unprofessional reference. Bad-mouthing another veterinarian or veterinary practice rarely pays. Know why your practice is special, and speak directly of the benefits of your practice and your delivery system. Be proud of what you stand for in the community.

• **Probe for more information.** Assess what was said, why it was said, and by whom. Was the source a client objection to something done in your practice? Do you need to perform damage control, or is it totally unfounded (remember, perceptions are real!).

• **Inform your staff.** Credible proof only cancels out erroneous information if the staff *knows* the facts and can deliver the information with pride.

• **Share the good news.** Let your service speak for itself. Don't be afraid to speak up and "correct the record," but do it based on your own honesty and dedication to the animals of the community.

69. What do we put into the new patient's "goody bag"?

The new patient and new client need to become bonded to the practice, but giving away "things" is not the most effective starting point. However, the animal may need a nutritional adjustment, and if the food is explained in terms of expected outcome, then a sample may be shared *after* the client education.

If the community has an endemic flea, parasite, or heartworm problem, the clients need to understand what that means, including the zoonotic implications. After they understand the issues, they can be given handouts so they will have a ready reference at home.

If they plan to travel with their pet, and you have determined when, how, and where, a protection plan can be developed and appropriate handouts offered for their travel files. Include Lyme disease information for trips to the Northeast, valley fever for the Southwest, salmon disease for the Northwest, endemic parasites for the Southeast, etc. Maps are always helpful!

A magnet that shows animal control, poison control, and your veterinary practice phone numbers is likely to be prominently displayed on the client's refrigerator.

70. How does participation in civic activities affect my practice's profits?

Social contacts are so important that the American College of Healthcare Executives *requires* community activity participation to keep a diplomate status. They have found that a healthcare facility must have a grass roots basis in their community to be effective in establishing a market niche in the consumer's mind.

If you do not have many social contacts, join at least two local associations or organizations. They are a valuable venue to meet and network with others who come into contact with your clients. Leverage your membership by choosing activities that help you meet people easily, give you visibility, and showcase your character and competence. Pour your energy into making conversational connections, share your business card at every opportunity, and offer your practice resources (e.g., speakers, tours) to others who have an interest in what you do.

71. How do I get my new doctor (receptionist team) to sell our products?

In veterinary healthcare delivery, the only thing we "sell" is peace of mind; all else the client is "allowed to buy."

Some see selling as a competitive situation; arm them with self-assurance that your practice is special for the patients. Others are self-conscious about the cost; focus them on the client's concern and the animal's welfare. Still others are self-centered and do not believe in the product or service for their own reasons; help them listen hard to the client's concern and respond to the client's needs and requests *before* they add their own bias.

Concentrate on the accomplishments of the practice. Flaunt the strengths of the individuals on your staff. Be proud of the equipment capabilities in the hands of your practice's providers.

72. I think we are "breaking client bonds" too often; what can we do better?

Broken promises come in many forms, from honoring the appointment to calling a client at the time agreed upon. Broken promises are a foundation for broken client bonds. There is a social contract that is embraced in all healthcare delivery, and it starts with "Do no harm" and continues to "Do what is needed." If the client perceives pain, or feels too much pressure to buy something they did not ask for, the client bond is weakened.

Clients come to a practice stressed, and instead of the practice paying attention to them, they are put into a "holding pattern." They feel ignored. Slighting a stressed client is often cause for that person to try another veterinary practice.

Be careful of telling a client that a computer will not allow it, that it is against hospital policy, or other forms of arguments. While a client may not always be right, they are seldom wrong! Do not blame a client; do not argue with a client—just ask, "What can we do to make it right?"

The high-tech world has caused some practices to put an eletronic sorting device between themselves and clients (those stressed people telephoning your practice). Ensure a real person answers and listens *before* a client is put into the electronic world of voice mail or electronic routing.

Client bonding is very similar to pricing; if the client believes he or she received more value than what was spent, it was a bargain. If a client felt important to the practice and known by the practice team, then the value increased in the client's mind, and the bond was enhanced.

2. HUMAN RESOURCES

RECRUITMENT OF THE RIGHT STAFF

1. Where do I find great staff members?

Great staff members are made, not found! Hire for **attitude** and train for the needed skills. Hiring for attitude means the resume is a screening tool, and the candidate needs an introductory period (60–90 days) to be trained to 85% competency for the job description duties.

Use a staff-based hiring team, consisting of a receptionist, nurse, caretaker, and manager/associate doctor, to screen and select the candidate. This is the same group that becomes the training team, which ensures that they accept accountability for the hiring criteria after the introductory period: **job competency** and **team fit**. Both must be present; if not, the person is released "at will."

The immediate need for people often causes the hire of a warm body, but that will never build a quality team. After the introductory period, continuous quality improvement requires continuous training, both in-service and external continuing education. In technical positions, continued growth using the newly available "distance-learning" programs should be a fringe benefit of employment. Training is necessary, to keep up with the rapidly changing knowledge base in the veterinary profession.

Great staff members are on great healthcare delivery teams, and great teams require great leaders. No one ever "managed" a horse to water. (And if you lead a horse to water, but it won't drink, as a veterinarian you can apply a stomach tube and make it drink!)

2. Where do I find "great-attitude" people?

The astute human resource recruiter *always* is looking for the "next person." For example, if the check-out person at the local grocery store (or a restaurant worker) is personable, give him or her a card and say, "If you ever want out of the retail clerks union (or food service business), we have a client relations position that may be of interest. Give me a call."

In the search for potential technicians, who really are nurses, local nurse aide vocational-tech programs can be offered at your hospital for in-service experience. Some will stay. Nurses aides already are committed to emptying bed pans, so veterinary hospitals are heaven by comparison!

Approved distance-learning programs are now available on the Internet (certified veterinary technician programs). You can make them and the "technician degree" available as a fringe benefit of employment.

3. What are the first steps when running a help-wanted ad?

Always start with a clearly worded **job position description** *before* writing the ad. Most jobs are redesigned between incumbents, and posting this description allows the adjustment to be accepted by the staff before the candidate arrives.

The ad should clearly request the type of initial contact desired; phone, fax, e-mail, or drop-off resume. Then the hiring team/manager follows up with an interview by phone in 24 to 48 hours. Establish the questions for the **phone screening** at the same time you place the ad. Often the name in the ad is not a real name, but a "special name" to alert the person answering the phone that an applicant is calling. You can hear them speak and respond to questions before you decide whether you want to invite them in for an interview. Consider letting your staff handle these screening calls for you. Let them select candidates for interview.

Have the staff form a three-person hiring team (manager plus receptionist, nurse technician, and animal caretaker) to interview the initial applicants (see *Building the Successful Veterinary Practice: Innovation & Creativity* [Volume 3] for interview questions and hiring team methods).

4. What are the components of a good job description?

A good job description helps staff candidates understand why they are there and what the practice expects from their on-the-job performance. It should include the following elements:

- Always start the job description by stating clearly that the staff members are there to serve clients and pets.
- Describe the responsibilities for the position in terms of "outcome expectations," rather than specific tasks.
- Some practices like to add "and other duties as needed and required" to the initial job description, but that phrase needs to be replaced by—
    See the challenge, solve the problem.
    See the need, make the change.
- Cite the standards of performance as "terms of employment," including dress, punctuality, overtime, expectations of assistance to others, and client confidentiality.
- Always have the benefits written as clearly as the job expectations, so that the orientation approach is balanced.

A good job description embraces the core values of the practice and shows the "training commitment" to a new candidate for the introductory period. The time-line for the introductory period should be adjusted for individual capabilities and learning rate, as determined by the practice training team. Traditionally, the period is 30 to 90 days.

5. How can I be more competitive in attracting and keeping good employees?
Don't forget that you have more than money to offer. Provide a professional environment and meaningful, satisfying work. The three Rs of staff employment are **respect, responsibility, recognition.** Offer flexible scheduling, including job sharing rather than part-time positions; this may be more important than money to many job candidates, and your practice is more competitive with these options.

Offer unique "perks," such as allowing staff members to bring their pets to work and veterinary pet insurance. Unlike the discounts of old, pet insurance increases the business tax deduction while increasing the cash return.

6. What key actions can I take to make my practice more efficient and improve productivity?
Four of the most overlooked areas are:
- Use technicians as "doctor extenders" so that you can see more patients in your practice.
- Improve your inventory management by improving the number of turns. Try to turn your inventory 8–12 times per year to maximize profitability.
- Match your practice hours to the hours in your community to make it easier for pet owners to make and keep appointments.
- Try high-density scheduling to maximize the number of patients you see each hour.

MOTIVATION VERSUS INCENTIVES

7. How do I best motivate the staff?
Motivation is not external; it comes from within. The traditional manager causes fear in an employee, but a leader creates an environment in which people can pursue their personal interests and desires in accordance with the practice's core values.

The practice culture should **nurture innovation and creativity** and require people to accept accountability for improving whatever is in their sphere of influence on a continuous basis. Continuous quality improvement (CQI) is based on each individual looking for things to improve as part of their daily environmental adjustment.

Many hospital surveys show that healthcare workers usually rank money in the top six workplace benefits, but never in the top three. The top three factors for improving the workplace environment generally are: respect, responsibility, and recognition.

8. How do I get them to buy into the practice programs?

Basic fact: behavior is a term of employment. Require *behavior*, not attitude (you hire for attitude). Address the behavior expected, not the personality or past performance.

Carefully consider before expressing anger or taking sudden action. Don't tell them what *not* to do. Clearly state what behavior and end goal is expected, and commit the resources so they can get there.

When identifying a program, clearly explain the outcome and the "why" of the patient advocacy or client-centered service. Use a brainstorming or **mind-mapping** session to allow the team to adjust and "tweak" the structure and specifics until the program becomes something special in their minds. (Mind-mapping starts with one core concept and expands as you jot down as many wild and crazy ideas as possible in the shortest amount of time.)

9. How do I sell a practice program?

Great programs are great sales promotions. In sales, **endorsements** are important. Always have great success stories available. Also have compassionate and caring stories of the consequences of not supporting the program. A good example is the graphic description of the wasting-away and pain that a cat endures during the terminal stages of FeLV. The mental picture must be so vivid that the cost and difficulties of the test and vaccination are inconsequential in the minds of the staff and clients.

Require each member of the key staff to accept accountability for one element of the program that they can accept and endorse. Give the "program sell" your very best, in terms of quality healthcare and patient advocacy. Employees seldom "buy in" when a program is presented only in economic terms.

10. What will encourage the team to execute a new practice program?

First, it must be presented as something special. There is an art to presentation. In advertising, it's called **"sell the sizzle,"** which comes from the television ads that display sizzling bacon, implying the aroma and flavor, but never addressing the cholesterol-laden fat of an animal that wallows in mud.

Start the program with excitement, and test it on the fly. Never try to predict all the problems before starting—it will never get started. Instead have a plan A and a plan B, and maybe even a C, D, and E, and expect the program to be tweaked daily by the team.

Stay centered on the outcome, and avoid process dissection. Get a "buzz" going on the team involvement and progress, not the speed bumps in the road. Start to brag about people and their efforts, and celebrate the participation (process) as well as the success (outcome).

11. How do I measure outcome success for staff executing a program?
Measures of success:
- being able to let go of leadership
- replication of effort at multiple levels of the practice
- "word-of-mouth" client-referrals
- the program becoming "mainstream" in the veterinary community
- the staff saying, "That's the way we do things around here!"

12. What can I do to change my boredom and/or fear of failure?
One of the authors (Catanzaro) has been doing volunteer leadership training with Jack Metcalfe (Boy Scouts of America) in Belize for almost a decade:

On the last trip, while Metcalfe was writing in his daily journal, he looked over and said, "Do you know what we were doing this day 3 years ago?" He said that we had been almost in the same location, encouraging Belize staff members to adopt what was to them a revolutionary method. This made me realize that Jack's daily journal was a quest of major proportions.

This example captures the essence, the passion, the imperative of the "program." **Effort really matters**, and everyone has a part.

Boredom simply is doing the same thing over and over until it requires no thought, and then the mind goes elsewhere. That is mundane life, and in more recent years has been labeled "burn out."

Fear of failure has been bred into most healthcare providers by licensure laws, but the fact is that most of the exciting programs are not licensure issues. They are mental: they start a fire in your belly and make others sit up and take notice.

The common denominator is: pursue something that really matters to you! Pursue it with drive, gumption, and imagination! Pursue something that counts in your internal value system! Something that defines you or the moment and is imbued with energy and a life of its own.

13. What type of incentives add to the CQI environment and staff harmony?

"Open-book management" concepts are a good foundation, but must be adjusted for a veterinary practice. Staff members know what is deposited each day, but they don't know the expenses. Think about the following "recognition" ideas (bonus and incentive are inappropriate terms for healthcare workers):

• Guarantee the staff salary as a percentage of gross (start with historical levels). Extra monies left at the end of each quarter are divided between staff members who have a full quarter of participation (40% of savings distributed immediately, 30% held for holiday surprise, and the balance held for Uncle Sam's tax requirements).

• Know the quarterly cost of drugs and medical supplies, but don't mix in diagnostic supplies, nutritional products, or boutique items. Take drug and medicine costs as a percentage of gross, and share 20% of the savings with the inventory management team when they reduce inventory costs.

• The nutritional counselors, who manage the nutritional inventory, also should track the net for their product lines. Quarterly they can be paid 20% of the earnings over 30% net.

CREATIVITY AND INNOVATION

14. How do I jump-start my team's creativity engine?

Require staff members to **bring one new idea** to any group meeting as their "admission ticket." The idea should focus on some aspect of their job and how they can improve what they do. The other staff members must seek the positive aspects of the idea *before* critiquing it.

Ask for two alternatives whenever confronted with a challenge (problem), and don't jump in with a solution. Don't allow staff to put their brains in your in-box; instead of "it can't work" or "it can't be done," ask for ways to make something else work to reach the desired outcome.

Expect staff to try to **make one improvement** in their work each day, focusing on the areas within their control.

When hearing new ideas, change the mind-set of the group from "Yes, but . . ." to "Yes, *and* . . . ." Work to continue where the last person left off. Get total commitment and team "buy-in" by *expanding* ideas, not limiting them.

Guarantee creativity by setting **idea quotas:** one minor evolutionary invention for every 10 days of work, and one major revolutionary brainstorm idea every quarter. Hold an **idea lottery** each month—each new idea gets a coupon good for the monthly staff meeting drawing of a special prize!

Create a **creativity corner**, where people can go to think new and wondrous things. Add an erasable white board for brainstorming, so that ideas and mind maps can grow from a group effort. Add pictures, decorations, and media resources that provide innovation fuel.

Make generating ideas fun and fearless. Stage a **stupid idea week** and hold a contest. Encourage camaraderie and be aware that "stupid" ideas often lead to great ideas. Post entries on the bulletin board and conduct an awards ceremony each day at lunch, with daily winners being entered in the drawing at the end of the week at a celebration luncheon.

Turn a staff hallway wall into a **hall of fame**. Exhibit photos and examples of specific staff members and their great idea(s).

15. How do I start the practice brainstorming?

It's a collective effort, so the innovation engine must be fueled before you start. **Rule one** is: everyone must hear the caring intention in whatever is said, so that people feel safe to share ideas. Divergent think is required; thus, collective confidence is required. **Rule two** is: anyone can disagree, but *never* make the other person wrong. Use the "Yes, *and* . . ." response instead of the "Yes, but . . ." or "No way . . ." reply.

The actual process has five informal steps. It's a free-flowing process, so don't get too structured.

Step 1—Problem Statement/Orientation of the Topic. Use outcome words, such as, "We are seeking new ways to . . ." or "We are looking to develop . . . ."

Step 2—Idea Generation. The best way to get a great idea is to work from 100 alternatives and discard those not needed. Each session needs both a facilitator and a recorder to keep the session freewheeling. A round-robin, in which individuals add to the idea and expand the thought process, often is improved by having everyone close their eyes so that they are less inhibited.

Step 3—Discussion and Evaluation. The recorder posts the ideas and then they are grouped, with pros and cons added, all without reference to who contributed or why. Solutions often lie within the synthesis of ideas and approaches.

Step 4—Decision and Implementation. The group picks the best alternative, and the details are written down for all to see. We recommend the mind-mapping format for this, since it is far more flexible than the traditional outline format. Develop and record a Plan A and a Plan B; outcome success measurements also are identified at this time. Establish a time line for implementation, and identify accountable individuals to coordinate and report on the process and outcomes.

Step 5—Assessment and Evaluation. While working Plan A, speed bumps likely will appear. Sometimes they are steep challenges—in fact, over 60% of the ideas in healthcare cannot be completed as initially designed. The project/idea coordinator can pull alternatives from Plan B and boost the process without any concern for checks and balances. There must be a 90-day implementation latitude before veto or final evaluation by supervisors; ideas must be given time to ripen on the vine. Trust the people you put in charge of the change garden and allow them to cultivate the innovation and creativity crop for the good of the practice.

16. I feel alone when making changes and decisions. How do I combat that feeling?

Build a network among creative friends from your place of worship, Rotary, and/or civic groups. This effort may be supplemented by hiring a consulting firm, attending university courses, enrolling in Dale Carnegie or Toastmasters, or even attending a short course on a topic of interest. Use all the brains you can find, beg, or borrow.

17. What if I am "blocked" creatively?

Re-frame your perspective, which often means looking at something upside down or inside out, or simply knocking down the roadblocks of bias and experience. **Creativity is a lifestyle**, so start by driving to work a different way, and go home by a second route. Eat at a new restaurant; shop at a new store; visit a new grocery and buy a food you have never eaten before.

Look at the "people roadblocks" in your mind and find a new route. Each person is an untapped resource: look at his or her strengths. Consider each person, yourself included, as someone who has something to share or has not been given the opportunity to try something new lately.

Overcome fear of rejection/failure by accepting that others have no power over your ideas. There is little risk sharing them; the worst someone can do is not be interested. Consider every meeting as an encounter between two comfort zones. If there is no click, it just means that the two comfort zones are not ready to be compatible.

Idea barriers can be physical, mental, and logistical. Don't let some obstacle stop you from exploring new horizons—just find a route around the barrier. The Internet is a new way of brainstorming in safety, since you can cruise the information highway and see other people's efforts without being recognized. You may even enter into a "chat room" and explore new ideas with total strangers . . . some find this fun, and most find it encouraging.

DISCIPLINE MATTERS

18. What is the best method for modifying inappropriate behavior?
Before you discipline an employee, ask yourself:
- Was the appropriate training provided?
- Was the staff member allowed to try the project/procedure under the supervision of a mentor and coached until comfortable with the skill?
- Did "recycling" occur when a person stumbled in the process, and were clear outcome expectations re-established?
- How was the recognition system used to show the right track?

Expectations should be clearly communicated. A veterinary team must depend upon each other and know what is expected, for patient welfare and client peace of mind. Everyone should understand that "letting down" another staff member is inappropriate behavior.

Hire people for team fit and personal competencies (culture, skills, and knowledge). Repeated failure in these areas is grounds for de-hiring!

19. How do I discipline a repeat offender?
"First" mistakes indicate that the employee is trying new things and learning. People who make no mistakes usually are striving for mediocrity. Encourage first mistakes!

If someone cannot learn, consider restructuring the job. A square peg does not fit into a round hole, but fits the square hole very well. Not all people can fill the shoes of the previous person, so plan to restructure jobs on a recurring basis, so individuals can "shine" in their own areas of expertise.

In a healthcare environment, if you cannot train a person to a level you can trust, release the person from employment to find a job with a better fit. Replace discipline efforts with an active search for someone who can do the job right!

20. What is the best way to deter tardiness?
Tardiness is an occasional event of life. Repeated tardiness is a discourtesy to other staff and cannot be tolerated. Describing tardiness as a team discourtesy, and not a time-clock issue, increases staff support. When someone arrives late, there are three general methods of addressing the issue (and it must be addressed *immediately*). The order here is flexible:
- State the hospital policy and the behavior required. Establish an agreement of consequence for repetition.

- Take the person aside and ask directly, "Why are you late?"
- Look at the person, lower your voice, and ask, "Is everything okay?"

POLICY MANUALS

21. Do I need a policy manual for my employees?

All business operations need an employee manual. A good employee manual ensures that human resource management is equitable. Generic manuals are available from most computer software vendors, and veterinary-specific ones are available from veterinary practice consultants (e.g., www.v-p-c.com) and other veterinary organizations and associations.

When you initiate a quest for a personnel manual, consider the core values of your practice and assess: vacation days, continuing education, sick days, healthcare benefits for staff and for staff animals, disability insurance, holidays, administrative leave, personal days, personal protective equipment/uniforms, duty hours, shift work, job sharing, and other routine issues.

22. Got any tips for modifying an employee manual?

Here's an important tip: job descriptions are not final! Every job description is a commitment to training. It should list the minimum standards expected. Establish a training system to ensure that employee competencies are reached within the first 90 days of employment. Once the training is "completed," the last element of the job description (usually "other duties as assigned") is changed to read: **see the challenge, solve the problem; see the need, make the change.**

Standard operating procedures or protocols must start with a **doctor's consensus**. Without clear protocols for services, the staff never become veterinary extenders, which means their ability to produce net is greatly decreased. Kal Kan Foods, Inc. sold a great "starting point" manual for less than $10 (over 200 pages) in the 1990s. You may have to look around for copies, but they are well worth it. Break out the sections to the staff members, small bites only, and have them rewrite the sample to meet what is happening in their world. Ideally, someone working from their rewrites can be 80% competent.

An operating manual is simply a starting point, since a veterinary practice is a series of problems waiting to be solved. Do not handcuff the staff in pursuit of protocols. Remember the phrase added to the job description at the end of the 90-day orientation training, and don't just talk the talk, but walk the walk.

TRAINING ISSUES

23. Is 90-day orientation training really needed for experienced people?

Yes. The orientation should allow the candidate to experience all elements of the practice during a nonproductive period (usually 2 weeks); then shadow all employees already working in the area to which he or she is assigned (usually another 2 weeks); then start working with and shadowing someone (usually 2–4 weeks). Finally, the new employee goes solo (until the end of the orientation/probationary period).

Training starts as a directive process: "These are our standards." The standards are based on core values and are inviolate: "Accept these standards or leave now." After the directive stage of training for skills and knowledge, the candidate must be "persuaded" that he or she is capable. After a first try doing the task or procedure, "coach" the candidate so that proficiency and confidence are gained. Delegation can occur only after this training triad: **direction-persuasion-coaching**.

Once the candidate is selected to join the healthcare team, orientation training is replaced by monthly in-service training, which is coordinated by staff for staff. Training should address one major issue each month to ensure that the entire staff—front, back, and inbetween—as well as doctors are on the same wavelength.

24. What are good appraisal techniques for enhancing performance?

In school, appraisals are past-tense test scores, with a bell curve of performance expectations. In healthcare, excellence is the standard, and grading on a curve is contrary to quality healthcare delivery.

Appraisals are moment-by-moment learning experiences based on quality and excellence in healthcare delivery. **Performance planning** (personal one-on-one commitments to change and to education in the upcoming 90 days) must become the method of choice for enhancing performance. Performance planning concepts require that the measurement of success be established between learner and mentor at the beginning of the 90 days. Advancement toward this goal is what you appraise at the end of the 90 days.

25. Is in-service training required in any state/province?

Only human healthcare has mandated in-service training. Veterinary medicine typically has focused on healthcare delivery techniques, rather than the staff development needed to get the outcome desired. If you accept the current professional standard that veterinary medical knowledge is doubling every 24 months, then in-service training is *essential* to practice growth.

Many distributors and vendors provide product training (and pizza) to practices they support. The American Veterinary Medical Foundation (AVMF) of the AVMA has established a new six-times-a-year video training program for practice teams called ClientLink. The AVMA also has published a series of client relations texts and handouts. AAHA has published a series of multi-media tools for staff development, and many independent vendors have developed and are offering training programs. Note that you must review and integrate any outside program before it can be used effectively as an in-service development tool.

26. How do we make the time for in-service training and other meetings?

Time is never "made"; it is only scheduled and sequenced effectively.

Think of the logger who must produce at ever higher levels of production, but never takes the time to sharpen his ax during the day. Production drops over time. The logger who routinely undertakes brief sharpening efforts maintains a sharper ax; cutting is easier, fatigue is less, and production is improved. It is the same in every mind, in every practice: a few, short (20-minute), individualized training efforts keep the skill level honed and sharp!

Trainers can go to the individual and grab a few moments one-on-one as the situation allows. If the trainers are rotated, a new staff member receives the current level of knowledge across all aspects of the job position.

27. How should training be organized?

Each trainer should be developed with new ideas and skills (train the trainer!), so that he or she can expand the knowledge base of the balance of the team. The "mentor and movie" method can work well in a busy practice. To use it, you'll need to obtain training tapes from Animal Care Training (ACT) tel. 1-800-357-3812. AAHA or another source can help teach your staff the general rules about OSHA and other safety issues, client care, patient care, and more.

Make up a list of all the things the new person has to learn. Divide the list according to the different sections of the hospital. Designate a mentor from each section to work with the new person and teach them the items on the respective section of the checklist. This method divides the responsibility for training more equally among staff members. It helps the new person get to know the other team members and to understand how work flows through the hospital.

SETTING UP THE SCHEDULE

28. How do I schedule people so that everyone is happy?
- Rule one: schedule the hospital, rooms, and tables—not people.
- Rule two: allow people to select shifts based on hospital needs, not individual needs.
- Rule three: people who do not want to work do not have to be employed.
- Rule four: equitable scheduling does not require everyone to be "happy."
  - Addendum: evening and weekend work may warrant a pay differential to recognize people who sacrifice personal desires for client needs.

29. What does "schedule the hospital" really mean?
One doctor works two consultation rooms when on outpatient duty. There is one nurse and one nurse assistant supporting the doctor, so that the two rooms can be simultaneously operated, but not "out-of-sync." The first 10 minutes in one room overlaps with the last 10 minutes in the other consultation room.

The inpatient nurse and inpatient doctor handle all emergencies, walk-ins, and drop-offs, allowing the outpatient team to stay on schedule. The inpatient doctor prioritizes the treatment room "white board" first thing every morning so the inpatient staff knows what is needed and in what order. For instance, grade 1 and grade 2 dentistries can be done while the inpatient doctor is doing surgery; but grade 3 dentistries require x-rays and possible extractions, so the doctor should not be scrubbed into surgery when those procedures are being done.

After lunch, the morning inpatient doctor shifts to outpatient, and the morning outpatient doctor shifts to inpatient to finish admitted cases. The late doctor comes in at noon, does 3 hours of spay/neuter and other predictable time surgeries, then does 4:30 to close outpatient (still two rooms per outpatient doctor).

30. How can I get control of my day at work?
The most important thing you can do is plan it realistically. For instance, plan a time to take and make telephone calls, and plan for interruptions. Schedule your appointments with free periods to allow you to catch up on records and make up for extra time spent on a complicated case, unforeseen delays, emergencies, and interruptions. Plan time to get out for lunch, take exercise breaks, meet with your staff, and do anything else that is important to you.

MILLENNIUM MANAGEMENT

31. Veterinary practices are scrambling to find clients and keep net income. What's happening, and what can we do?

The rules are changing, and the old methods don't work. Vaccination and pet population income is waning, pet populations have stabilized, and the number of store-front practices has increased in most metroplex communities. Practices must accept these changing environmental factors.

Be the first practice to use **new healthcare delivery ideas**, such as nursing appointments, high-density scheduling, more visits at lower average client transaction rates, alternative medicine, VIP resort suites for pet guests, and behavior management advisors.

Develop a **strategic foresight**. Make assumptions on the community's future using the best information from the city planners, chamber of commerce, rotary contacts, church sources, and other merchants and civic leaders.

Look at a **team redesign**. Include new duty area accountabilities, target outcomes, and client-centered services. Ask clients what is needed to make them return more often with *all* of their family pets.

Feed the innovation engine residing in the minds of every staff member, every client, and every community contact. Look at things upside down and inside out to find the unusual approach to being unique in the community.

32. How do we rise to the challenges of the new millennium?
- Reconnect to the values that motivate staff and doctors.
- Target retention and training of the best staff available; don't underpay!
- Start with a quality healthcare delivery perspective, then look at costs.
- In larger practices, focus on educating governance (i.e., Board of Directors, etc.) to handle policy and precedent, while empowering providers and staff to deliver operational excellence.
- Know what the community residents want. Ignore the "national averages," and set your own goals to improve convenience, increase client education, and ensure continuous quality improvement against your own standards.
- Design the "delivery system of the future" by mixing styles of medicine with retail that fits how people live. Help people understand that they cannot have more benefits and choices without paying a higher price.

33. Is the new millennium really that unique?

In the past century, manufacturing of "things" made America special. The third-world countries copied this trend, and reduced the impact of American products on the world.

In the coming century, knowledge is all that America can really broker. We have the educational and developmental edge to make a difference in the world market of information sharing.

Client awareness is developed by environmental influences. The undercurrent of veterinary practice in the past century was selling things. The driving force in the new millennium will be **brokering knowledge**.

34. The words we use set the tone of the practice. What are the new words for the new millennium?

The words you use shouldn't be just buzz phrases . . . you must walk the walk!

New Words	Old Words
A performance	A job
Act of commitment	Puttin' in the time
Memorable	Close enough
Wow, gee whiz!	Blah
Team members	Employees
A signature piece	It has always been this way
Epitome of character	Faceless
Innovation and creativity	Predictable and safe
Mastery of excellence	Acceptable work
Exhausting effort	Numbing existence
Talent rules	Hierarchy habits
Adventuresome	Risk-averse
Growth experience	Another day
It matters!	No big deal . . .

35. What is the secret to success in the new millennium?

Steve Heller described the pioneer American designer, Paul Rand: "He took every opportunity to redefine a project in brief so that the problem could be solved according to his own vision." George Bernard Shaw said, "The reasonable man adapts himself to the world; the unreasonable man persists in trying to adapt the world to himself. Therefore all progress depends on the unreasonable man."

The secret is an internal focus of excellence, doing the usual as if it was unusual, or doing the unusual as if it was usual, if you want to be remembered:

- Take the task at hand, any task, and turn it into something that makes a difference in the minds of others; say it, shout it, live it!
- Reward those with an excellent failure.
- Starve those striving for mediocre successes.

36. What are the critical elements of the creativity process?

This question is the first step in killing creativity . . . it cannot become routine! Better question: What can I do to create the environment needed?

• Write the current project description in less than one page, fax or e-mail it to three "free-thinking" people outside the practice, and ask them to help you rethink the issues.

• Get three teammates together, *today*, for at least an hour offsite, and brainstorm a new version of the project based on the desired outcomes rather than the process or people.

• Talk to the strangest people you know, the youngest, the oldest, or even the weirdest, and ask them to reinvent the issues and assumptions, as well as the direction of the effort.

• Re-examine cultural assumptions, community pressures, and the boss' preferences in terms of, "What will excite them?"

• Stay curious to the very end, then seek new perspectives as you get comfortable. Don't get bored, and don't accept the mundane as routine.

37. What do creative thinkers have in common?

Thomas Edison, Ben Franklin, Leonardo da Vinci, Virginia Woolf, Carl Jung, and even Charles Darwin kept **daily journals**. They understood that new ideas often come from combining many disparate pieces of information or concepts over an extended period of time.

The great business leaders, e.g., the CEOs of all Fortune 500 companies, have **written goals**. The simple act of writing a goal allows a commitment to become a reality rather than a wish.

Work from the front of your journal to the back (a loose-leaf binder is better); you do not need to be chronological. Have a list of "Awful Stuff" in the back, and a list of "Gee Whiz–Cool Stuff" in the front. Build a **mind map** for each new idea.

Start by visiting a mall today. Observe the stores, people, and merchants; then add ten things to each list (Awful vs. Gee Whiz) and at least one new mind-map idea. Apply at least four observations, good or bad, to the project of the moment.

38. Can I use benchmarking in this new millennium quest for innovation?

"Benchmarking" is a 1990 corporate term for brain-picking. Brain-picking is simply using all the brains you can beg, borrow, or steal. It involves applying others' impressive ideas to your own projects.

Benchmarking has been used by some veterinarians and veterinary managers as an excuse not to change, because they only look inside the veterinary profession and do not see anything new or exciting. The idea is to look *outside* a specific industry for new ideas that worked in other industries or professions.

Life is brimming with new, stimulating experiences. It takes a little nerve and a trust that your team will be able to "adjust on the fly" to make the idea work better each day.

3. STAFF TRAINING AND ORIENTATION*

1. Why is staff training important?

The success of any program or promotion depends on the people who are responsible for carrying out the details: they must be educated about what they are expected to do. This is the core definition of training—**educating the force about expectations.**

Remember, training is an ongoing process; it'll never be completed or over. Just like housekeeping or even medical record documentation, it'll always require updating, refining, and implementation.

An abundance of evidence supports the belief that a well-trained workforce is more productive, happier, and more stable (less turnover) than a comparable group of people without clear directions or instructions. In that sense, training is not a detraction from the work at hand, but a means of performing the work better and more efficiently.

Practices that set aside time and resources for regular staff training not only are more profitable, but are simply nicer places to work because the staff is more focused.

Just as a practice must embrace new medical ideas and methods to stay competitive, it also must find ways to keep the staff up-to-date on issues and directives.

- The traditional workplace of "9–5 and closed for lunch" is no longer the norm in the veterinary profession, so traditional training methods like meetings and seminars are not the answer to every problem.
- Traditional methods still have a place in the training schedule, but alternative methods must be employed if the business is to stay ahead of the problems.

2. What is my role as leader in the training process?

Every training program is destined to succeed or doomed to fail according to the emphasis it gets from the leadership. If the practice owners relay and support the message that all training—medical, safety, and procedural—is a mandatory component of employment, then the staff will take is seriously. If the leadership doesn't show genuine support for training programs, the staff will be unenthusiastic about anything that is perceived as "more work" or that disrupts the normal day's events.

Leaders must also follow the rules that are in place for other workers.

---

* Also see Appendix C.

- The staff will not abide by the safety rules if the veterinarian owner of the practice believes in a "Do as I say, not as I do" philosophy.
- This goes for attendance at required training functions also!
- The presence and participation of the practice leaders sends the message that the issue is important.
- Likewise, the leaders' absence sends the message that this stuff isn't serious enough to get their attention, so it must not be very important.

Perhaps the best way for the leadership to support a training program is to make time in the schedule for it. Successful practices recognize that staffing at a level barely adequate to cover the workload on an average day leaves little room in the schedule for staff improvement. Staff meetings or training sessions after working hours or during other nonbusiness periods will be resented as intrusions into personal time. Additionally, the staff will get the impression that the message (training) wasn't important enough to take time away from the routine, so it's just another one of those boring, useless meetings. However, by conducting training on "company time," the business is sending the message that the topic is relevant and important.

Finally, the leadership must create the expectation that all staff members will participate and support the training. Associate veterinarians or senior technical staff members cannot be allowed to disrupt the timing or flow of the training. Routine treatments, telephone calls, and deadlines are important, but so is training, and neither should overshadow the other. Only the senior leadership of the hospital can make training as important as any other part of the practice.

3. When is the best time to train staff members?

Just as there are various stages of medicine, the same is true for adult learning: we are more likely to influence someone's decisions or habits early in the process, rather than later. Once the "problem" has taken hold, it is far harder to cure than it was to prevent in the first place. Exposing the staff to training early makes them more likely to develop the habits outlined in the training, and less likely to pick up "bad" habits from an existing staff member.

- When a new person joins the team, he or she is in a learning phase and not yet an indispensable employee.
- The longer the employment, the more responsibility is gained and, in most cases, the less receptive an employee is to changing habits.

Another reason to get the training done early is practicality. The newly hired staff member has the time to sit down and read detailed materials. Even after just a month on the job, it's unlikely that a staff member can (will?) find the time to examine the materials he or she would have during the first few days.

4. What is "remedial" training?

If the analogy of initial training is like general animal husbandry, then remedial training has to be like treating a disease. If you notice a staff member is not following the procedures, take immediate action before the situation worsens. The staff member must be corrected and, if necessary, re-trained on the correct procedures. Remedial training does not have to be as extensive as the initial training and can focus entirely on the parts that the staff member did not understand.

Although the goal of remedial training is to change undesirable habits, it should not be viewed as disciplinary action. However, if a staff member continues to violate the hospital policies even when they understand the training, then separate disciplinary action is appropriate.

5. Describe "in-service" training.

Continuing with the medical analogies, perhaps the easiest way to prevent problems is with regular vaccinations; that's exactly the same objective of in-service training. In-service training strengthens existing good habits with additional information or instructions, so that the staff member continually improves. In-service training should be viewed as the regular, on-going process of disseminating information within the hospital. It supplements existing knowledge or training for the existing staff member. In-service training can be conducted in a meeting format, but it often is just as effective via nonparticipatory methods such as technical bulletins, memos, or written directives.

In most practices, several staff members are engaged in the various training stages (early, remedial, in-service) at any given time—that's normal. One of the many jobs of the veterinary practice leader is to coordinate the various needs of each staff member with the needs of the practice. Only by understanding the different stages of training and their uses and objectives can you institute an effective training program in your practice.

6. What is the most effective method of training?

The **one-on-one style** of training is definitely the most effective when structured properly. This style allows lots of individual attention and gives the instructor immediate feedback on the student's progress.
- It must be structured. There must be a list of tasks to accomplish in a logical order.
- The down side of this style of training is obvious: time. The instructor must have the ability, inclination, and time to spend with the student.

- One-on-one is not the same as "Follow Jane around; she'll show you what you need to know." That's not training at all—it's simply throwing the person into the work and expecting eventual learning.

7. **Describe some other training styles.**

Veterinary practices use the **on-the-job style** of training most often because it is the best for making sure that the student learns the task a specific way. It can be the most permanent form of training, since the student continually practices what has been learned. Contrary to popular belief, this style often is the most difficult for a student. First, the student must be in the "learning mode." Many staff members are too preoccupied with accomplishing daily tasks or concerned about other problems to absorb the training. Second, unless the student understands the background of the task and the theories behind the steps, he or she will never really understand how to accomplish the goal. The steps are learned, but not the concepts, so when something goes wrong, there is no knowledge base to solve the problem. In such situations, the process stops, and the employee must obtain further instruction from the supervisor to continue.

Formal meetings are the method of choice for providing background or foundation-type knowledge. They also are the most effective at direct dissemination of information to large groups, such as daily briefings and updates on projects. Formal meetings usually are the best forum for in-service training on procedural matters.

Note that most gatherings of people quickly turn into "gripe sessions" if there is not an agenda and clearly stated purpose for the meeting. These sessions are difficult to coordinate in busy practices if the goal is 100% staff participation. You can record the meeting so that staff members who miss it (e.g., answering phones, vacationing) can receive the information.

Video/computer-based training is fast becoming the most popular style for the veterinary practice. The ability to stop the action and review the procedure as often as the student needs is a powerful benefit. Moreover, videos can be viewed individually by many staff members —without a major time investment by the supervisor or trainer. Note, however, that video and computer-based training lacks one critical element of learning: a person to ask questions of when something doesn't make sense. It is critical that any video/computer instruction be followed immediately by one-on-one time with a qualified instructor. Without this followup and interaction, the video is just an exercise and not a training tool.

Correspondence training is the use of written materials to disseminate information; it is helpful when issuing directives or making time-sensitive announcements. The most common form of correspondence training is the memorandum. Although this style of training lacks the personal interaction necessary for learning complex tasks, it is useful because it can be given to an unlimited number of students at the same time. Many practices use a "Monday Morning Memo" to clarify special happenings in the coming week and to keep a lid on the "rumor mill." Written training has one major drawback: the student must be motivated or forced to read it!

The biggest benefit of using **outside courses** to train staff members is the ability to capitalize on the talents of outside experts. Courses can be veterinary-specific (e.g., veterinary CE meetings) or can cover general business knowledge. Here's a tip: require the staff member(s) that attends the session to bring back the main ideas and present an in-service session to the rest of the staff.

Perhaps the best reward of outside courses is that the staff member has "ownership power" of the ideas and tasks. When people feel in control of their jobs, they usually are more productive and happy! Drawbacks of outside courses include scheduling and coverage conflicts that arise when a staff member is away from the practice.

8. What are the benefits of using a training schedule?

No matter what the task at hand, having an outline of the major milestones of the project certainly makes completing it easier. The same is true for continuing education and training. Practice leaders who take the time to prepare a training schedule are significantly more likely to accomplish their training goals than those who rely on their memory and the demands of the everyday workload to determine the topics.

Begin by asking each staff member if training has been adequate. If the answer is no, listen to any suggestions and respond accordingly. In this way, you get valuable information, and they get the satisfaction of knowing that they have been heard.

- Rank the topics by importance—the highest ranking topic will be the first one delivered; the lowest ranking will be at the end of the schedule.
- Assign just one or two topics to each training date, and post the schedule for everyone to see.
- Keep the schedule current. When you have to make changes or adjustments, indicate them on the written schedule so that everyone is up-to-date.

Assign staff members to be instructors for each topic. Be sure to task *all* staff members. The best way for someone to learn a topic is to teach it to someone else! Let your instructors know the date of the session and how long they should take to deliver the message. Give them resources on the topic (or point them in the right direction), and make sure they understand what the focus of the session should be.

Remember, planning is the key to success when it comes to training, and the first step is creating a schedule so that everyone knows the plan.

9. How do I make training replicable?

Do any of the following scenarios sound familiar?
- It's impossible to get everyone together at the same time.
- While we have meetings, someone has to answer the phones and assist clients at the reception area, or we have to close the hospital.
- As soon as we complete an extensive training or safety meeting, we add another staff member to the team who needs the same training.
- The problem with our traditional training programs is that they are too labor-intensive to deliver.
- Once the session is completed, the information is no longer available for later use.

Traditionally, veterinary training has been conducted in a meeting environment, with mixed results. The solution is to plan the training delivery method as well as you prepare the materials. The best method of replicating training is to videotape each session! Invest in a video camera with a stand, or rent one for individual meetings.

10. How do I videotape meetings?

Set the camera up so that the action specific to the training is captured on tape. If the training is for a specific procedure that requires a demonstration, then have someone "zoom in" on the technique when the time comes. If the meeting is going to be more verbal than hands-on, then a wide shot of the entire room is appropriate.

Check the sound levels and picture quality by taping a few minutes of "test" talking from the center of the room during the setup. Using a small external microphone plugged into the recorder instead of the built-in microphone greatly improves the sound quality. Be sure to label the tape with the topic of the meeting and the date.

There is a side benefit to this process: attendance at meetings usually increases because most people would rather attend the "real-time" sessions than have to view a recorded one.

11. Not every piece of information warrants videotaping. What are other methods of making training replicable?

Some information does not require formal training sessions or courses. Issuing directives, reiterating procedures, or simply reminding staff members of a message are all types of training that can be accomplished with **memos, notes, and signs.** As a general rule, no more than two "directives" should be circulating or posted at a time. Multiple memos are likely to confuse the staff, and they may just ignore all of them. Likewise, remove old messages from the bulletin board after all staff members have seen and initialed them. This action reduces clutter and gives the impression that the message is important.

Another method is the **practice training manual.** Get a three-ring binder and label it appropriately. When you take down a notice or when a memo has been initialed by everyone, put it in the binder along with all handouts, quizzes, and written information from real-time meetings. This way, there's always a record of what information was put out. Additionally, new employees obtain an "institutional memory," without actually having been present, by reviewing the training manual when they are first hired. The manual also helps when you have one staff member who just doesn't get it. He or she can review the handouts and session material without much additional time from the supervisor.

12. **List some important training tips.**
    - Establish a form of feedback for every session, so that the leadership can be assured that the message was received as it was intended.
    - Direct the instructor to prepare a few short questions to administer as a quiz after the session.
    - The instructor can ask individuals to demonstrate a particular technique.
    - Always have some method of ensuring that the participants understood the training!
    - Keep a written record of attendance for every training session conducted.

13. **What are some secrets for running successful meetings?**
    One of the most common complaints from staff members and supervisors alike is the amount of time that is dedicated to "useless" meetings and training. It seems the larger the organization grows, the more accurate that complaint becomes. You can avoid this trap by following a few guidelines for effective meetings and in-service sessions:
    - Make sure the topic is **relevant** and **timely**. Use a recent situation or medical case to help illustrate the point of the training.
    - Make the information relevant by using **actual examples** whenever possible.
    - **Avoid "old news"** topics, unless there is a need for repetition or remedial instruction.

- Use **alternatives to meetings** whenever applicable. When you simply need to disseminate information, without evaluating opinion or performance, consider posting a memo on the bulletin board or including it in each staff member's pay envelope.
- Instead of the traditional "top down" training, some practices require each staff member to submit a suggestion for improvement or a summation of a journal CE article each month. This form of **self-directed learning** is gaining great acceptance in the business world as a supplement to interactive training topics. This method of instruction is individualized, and the entire organization spends less time in boring meetings. Note, however, that not all training topics are conducive to noninteractive methods.
- **Dedicate enough time** for the topic. Limit sessions to one or two topics and avoid the tendency to "get it all over with at once." As a general rule, shorter, more frequent sessions can be accommodated easier than longer ones; most people can find 30 minutes a week for an in-service session, but find it harder to "break away" for a full afternoon once a month.
- Retention of information and compliance with directives is greater when the message is delivered in shorter, more frequent formats.
- **Eliminate foreseeable interruptions.** Patient treatments, client phone calls, and special projects are important, but unless they are a true medical emergency, they should not be allowed to interfere with a scheduled meeting or training session.
- Let the senior staff members know that their full participation is expected, and they must schedule their day accordingly. Don't let one or two "indispensable" staff members disrupt the session for everyone else.
- Leave a skeleton crew at the front desk to take phone calls and assist clients. They can watch the videotape of the meeting later.
- **Concentrate on the positives.** Avoid the urge to use the training to reprimand for past mistakes. Focus on the correct way to do things, and save the reprimands for more appropriate times.
- **Start and stop on time.** Be conscious of everyone's schedule. Do not wait for the chronic "stragglers." It's better to close the meeting on time—even if all the information has not been discussed—than it is to extend the meeting.
- Except in very rare situations, the material that is not discussed can be disseminated by means of a handout or even a memo prepared after the meeting.

By following these simple suggestions, you can hold more informative, less disruptive meetings or training sessions. Remember that old adage: "The team that trains together stays together!" And who wouldn't want more harmony and less turnover in their staff?

14. How can I address nonattendance problems?

Make sure that the audience has had **plenty of notice.** One of the favorite excuses for missing training or other important sessions is "Nobody told me!" You can avoid this annoying excuse by planning the sessions well in advance. Try including a reminder note in each staff member's pay envelope (or attached to their new time cards) about a week preceding the event. Also post notices of important meetings on the bulletin board or near the time clock.

Make the training replicable by providing handouts and even videotaping the session. Thus, staff members who miss the actual session can still benefit.

Time the training to the work schedule. Establish a regular time and place for training. By having the training "built into" the schedule, you have a better chance of attendance, participation, and retention of the materials, because the staff does not view the session as a disruption to the normal work day. Ask the staff when it would be best for them. Strive for weekly or at least monthly sessions that are held the same day of the week at the same time of the day.

15. What is the best time for a meeting and/or training?

Retention of information and participation increases for meetings in the morning. Thursday seems to be the best day of the week for in-service sessions. Avoid Mondays, Fridays, lunch-time, late afternoon, and after-work sessions, when enthusiasm is at the lowest.

Finish orientation training of new staff members before you become dependent on their time. Large businesses have learned that if they schedule the new staff member for orientation on the first 2 days of employment, it will be accomplished, but if they wait until the staff member assumes duties, the success rate goes down dramatically. Use a checklist to ensure that all of the details are covered.

4. REGULATORY MATTERS

HEALTH AND SAFETY

1. How many employees must a business have before OSHA rules apply?

OSHA's standards apply to every nongovernmental business when there is at least one nonowner employee. OSHA standards do not apply to self-employed persons without employees; however, if the business employs at least one worker, then the standards apply to the entire business, including the owner.

2. What is the chance of my practice getting inspected by OSHA?

Since most OSHA inspections of veterinary practices are the result of complaints from employees or former employees, the risk is directly related to the employer/employee relationship. Of course, no one can predict when a complaint will be filed, but practices with leaders who take the staff's concerns seriously generally have fewer regulatory complaints than those who ignore the staff's concerns.

Note that the inspection is only part of the investigation; many investigations do not involve inspections.

3. Can OSHA inspect my practice at any time they choose?

Unless the OSHA inspector (Health & Safety Compliance Officers [HSCO]) has reason to believe that an "imminent danger" situation exists, the inspection must occur at a time and in such a manner so as to cause minimal disruption to the operation. Although not mandatory, the HSCO often calls the owner of the business and arranges a meeting time for the inspection. If the HSCO arrives for an unannounced inspection, the owner can request that the inspection be rescheduled at a more convenient time. If the owner uses this right as a delay tactic, the HSCO can obtain a court order allowing immediate access.

4. Can OSHA inspect my practice while I'm not there?

Under the Occupational Safety & Health Act, business owners (employers) have the right to be present or designate a representative to act on their behalf during any investigation or inspection. If the owner never leaves the facility, then there's no problem, but that's not practical for most businesses, including veterinary hospitals. Unless some precautions have been taken in advance, the owner may unintentionally waive that right in an inspection.

If an employee admits a HSCO to the facility for an inspection in the owner's absence, it usually is assumed that the employee has the authority to do so. Any evidence or statements obtained generally are used to determine the existence of a violation and to set the proposed fine.

Every business should identify those individuals who are authorized to act on behalf of the owner in his or her absence and provide specific guidance on the parameters of that authority. For example, the associate veterinarian may have the authority to make customer satisfaction decisions in addition to fulfilling the medical duties normally associated with that position; however, the associate veterinarian may be required to contact the owner prior to signing any binding agreement involving the practice. The same philosophy is true for regulatory compliance matters—define the parameters of authority for all staff members and put it in writing!

A component of each practice's Hospital Safety Manual should be a policy reflecting the owner's rights and the staff's authority during an inspection. This written statement is vital if the owner *does not waive* his or her right to be present during an inspection. It normally is enough to effect postponement of an inspection until the staff can contact the owner.

5. Do all OSHA investigations include an inspection?

No. Some investigations are handled via correspondence. OSHA sends a notice to the business and asks for information relevant to the investigation. If the business provides evidence that they are "doing things right," then OSHA is likely to forgo the onsite inspection. If, on the other hand, the business fails to respond or gives less than credible evidence, then an onsite inspection probably will occur.

6. What are the fines for violating OSHA standards?

OSHA publishes a set of "proposed" fines that almost always are followed in the initial citation. These fines start at about $1,000 per infraction for "less than serious" violations and significantly more for "serious" violations. There also are multiplication factors for special situations like repeat or willful violations. For instance, a serious violation that also is a repeat violation and, in the HSCO's opinion, a willful violation on the part of the employer can be fined as much as $70,000.

7. How do I find out about what standards apply to my practice?

OSHA Standards are published in the Code of Federal Regulations (CFR) in Chapter 29. You can obtain a copy of the CFR by (1) purchasing a printed copy from the U.S. Government Printing Office; (2) purchasing a CD-ROM version from the U.S. Government Printing Office or from several commercial vendors; (3) viewing, printing, or downloading copies from the OSHA web site (www.osha.gov); (4) purchasing a veterinary-specific OSHA compliance kit that "deciphers" the rules and gives implementation advice (check out the web site www.v-p-c.com/phil for examples).

8. How do I get my OSHA program started?

Decide if you want to do it yourself, or if you want to hire someone. Many practice owners and administrators believe the best way to achieve compliance with OSHA rules is to hire a professional to do it for them. Many consultants specialize in this service, and it is by far the easiest way to go. Prices are about $550–$1500, depending on the company and the breadth of the program.

Learn the requirements. Regardless of whether you want to implement the plan yourself or hire someone to do it for you, you should have a working knowledge of the requirements. Copies of every OSHA standard, directive, or interpretation can be found on OSHA's web site at www.osha.gov. The same material is available for purchase from the U.S. Government Printing Office (202/512-1800) on CD-ROM and in printed form.

9. What tools can help me with OSHA compliance?

The best solution for most practices is to purchase a **veterinary-specific compliance kit** or **newsletter subscription**. These tools will "decipher" the regulations into terms and procedures you can understand and implement. Subscriptions run about $30, and the compliance kits are approximately $75–$350. Note that compliance kits are simply an interpretation of the rules by the author. OSHA does not "approve" or "certify" any person or publication in this regard.

10. I've begun preparations. What is the next step?

Make an **implementation plan**—list changes required and procedures that need attention. Concentrate on one subject at a time, and work your way through the plan. It's okay to make adjustments and even rearrange the order of events on the plan when the need arises. Even if you are not completely finished with the implementation plan before you are inspected by OSHA, having it often is a critical factor in OSHA's determination of whether you show intent and progress toward compliance.

11. How can I organize my implementation plan?

Take it one step at a time. Start with the most hazardous jobs, and establish a procedure that must be followed when exposure to the hazard can occur. The plan always should be in writing and reflect what is actually done. The perfect plan is useless if nobody does it that way! Train the staff on the expectations, and *enforce* the plan. You may get some grumbling from a few staff members at first, but soon the new method becomes a habit.

Pay particular attention to the safety equipment required. Make sure that your equipment is appropriate for protecting the user and fits properly. A great example is the radiation protection gloves in most practices. Although they may be appropriate for the radiation present, if the staff members can't use them because they are too big, too small, or simply not flexible enough, they are inadequate.

12. The implementation plan is underway. Now what?

Create a **Hospital Safety Manual** (HSM). The best way to organize a hospital safety program is to put it all in one place. A one-resource compilation of all of the safety-related information in the practice gives the impression of a comprehensive program instead of a "hit-or-miss" one. The HSM is the primary means of communication on safety matters between the leadership and the staff; therefore, only include information that directly instructs or educates the employee. Instill the HSM as the official policy of the practice.

- Use a three-ring binder conspicuously labeled "Hospital Safety Manual."
- Use tabbed dividers to create sections, e.g., General Rules, Fire Prevention and Response, Anesthesia, Radiation, Accident Prevention, Infection Control, Chemicals, and Violence Prevention.
- Don't clutter the manual by including compliance instructions and similar materials designed for the manager.
- Include extracts of journal articles and related educational materials to further inform the staff on particular hazards and to reinforce the practice's safety policies.

13. Where should the Hospital Safety Manual be located?

Keep the HSM in a convenient location—usually in a "neutral" area like the break room, treatment area, or lab. Avoid keeping it in the doctor's or manager's office, because there may be some "situational intimidation" that would prevent a new or concerned worker from reviewing it. Make sure every staff member knows where the HSM is located and that they have a right to review it whenever necessary.

14. What details should I consider when polishing the implementation plan?

Train—train—train. Once you have researched the issue, evaluated your procedures, and written a plan, the only step that's left is to train the staff on the new or revised procedures. An effective training program doesn't have to be complicated or expensive. Simply set aside some time on a regular basis for the staff to review information relevant to their jobs, and make sure that safety measures are implemented.

Re-evaluate and adjust. Don't be afraid to make changes. Nothing ever works out exactly as planned, and you must be flexible. Ask the staff for input during the development phase; you may find that they have concerns you never realized. As you implement the various components of the plan, you'll learn easier and better ways to communicate your message. Don't be afraid to try new ideas or methods: if they work, you're finished; if they don't, then you've learned what not to do next time!

15. What is an MSDS?

Material Safety Data Sheets (MSDS) are produced by the chemical manufacturer to explain the specific properties of their product. The MSDS differs from a package insert because of the intended audience: a package insert is intended for the one-time or casual user of the product, whereas the MSDS focuses on the person who is exposed to that product on a regular basis. There is no mandated format or design that a manufacturer must follow when producing an MSDS, so don't be confused by the variety you'll receive. OSHA does mandate specific data or information to be present.

The most useful data on an MSDS for the veterinary worker are the Health Hazard, Protective Equipment, and Spill Clean-up and Disposal sections; the remaining sections are of marginal value in everyday operations, but are important in emergency situations or when investigating whether the product is involved in a suspected illness outbreak.

16. Where do I obtain an MSDS?

First, call the distributor who supplied the product. If the distributor or supplier can't get it for you in a reasonable time, contact the manufacturer. Often the manufacturer provides a phone number directly on the product's label.

Many manufacturers and distributors have put their MSDS on web sites. Many MSDSs also are available on a special CD-ROM produced by North American Compendiums, Inc. (tel. 800/350-0627).

17. What's the best way to file MSDS?

The MSDS should be filed in a systematic way. It is best to file them alphabetically by the product name, instead of by operational area or category. Use a three-ring binder (or two) with tabbed alphabetical dividers. This system presents less confusion to the staff member; e.g., is bleach filed under disinfectants or under housekeeping supplies? If a product is known by several names, you can place a piece of paper in the alphabetical file that directs the reader to look under the specified name given by the manufacturer (e.g., Lasix7—see furosemide).

Be sure to cover the filing system and understanding of MSDS during staff training sessions. The real test of the training's effectiveness is to ask any staff member (try the newest one) to retrieve a specific MSDS quickly.

18. Can I use a CD-ROM or the Internet for my MSDS library?

Yes. A CD-ROM with thousands of MSDS already formatted for easy retrieval is available; however, in most situations, the applicable MSDS must be printed on regular paper and filed.

At the present time, the best source of electronic veterinary-specific MSDS is COMPAS Software, distributed by North American Compendiums, Inc. (tel. 800/350-0627). This program has MSDS for most of the veterinary-specific products available today, as well as some hard-to-find ones for products that are no longer produced. Additionally, the hard copies printed by the computer program are in some ways better than the originals from the manufacturer. They typically print in fewer pages than the original, because of the type style and layout, and—perhaps more importantly—they are standardized! Vital information can be located quickly because it's in the same place for every MSDS.

For examples of website MSDS, see Vedco (www.vedco.com) and W. A. Butler (www.wabutler.com), as well as numerous generic sites that have basic chemical information available (e.g., www.hazard.com).

19. Do we really need an eyewash unit in the practice?

Yes. An eyewash station should be near any area of the hospital where corrosive chemicals are used. There is some flexibility in the rules, but do not expect employees to go up or down stairs, through multiple doors, or around an "obstacle course" of hazards to get to the device. Remember, the person who needs an eyewash can't see, so it has to be easy to find!

It is best to have an eyewash in every room where lab procedures are performed (e.g., with reagents or formalin), where photo developing chemicals are mixed or used, and where hazardous cleaning chemicals or insecticides are used. Locate the eyewash in a place where contamination from the chemicals in use is minimal. Be conscious of overhead cabinets or shelves and adjacent obstructions; ensure that an injured person can get his or her head and body into the correct position.

20. Is a hose or faucet acceptable as an eyewash?

No! The spray attachments for tubs and sinks also are inappropriate for eye flushing, because the water pressure is unregulated, and the streams of water from these devices usually are so fine that laceration of the cornea could occur.

Eyewashes are designed for two primary dangers: foreign body irritations and chemicals. **Foreign bodies** usually affect one eye, and once the object is removed, the flushing process can be discontinued. **Chemicals** usually affect both eyes simultaneously, and both must be thoroughly cleansed for a long time to remove any residuals of the chemical. The hand-held bottles of saline solution that sometimes are mounted in "stations" on the wall are designed for foreign body irritations; they are not intended for chemicals. They contain a limited amount of solution, and the worker can flush only one eye at a time. An effective eyewash provides an uninterrupted flow of water and flushes *both eyes simultaneously*.

21. What protective equipment must be worn by staff members when bathing animals or applying insecticides?

Follow the label directions and MSDS precautions for all shampoos, dips, and conditioners. These instructions specify exactly which articles of protective equipment must be used. Some of the newer, more natural products may only require protective eye wear, but more hazardous chemicals typically dictate the use of gloves, goggles, waterproof aprons, and even respirators.

As an alternative to the traditional grooming aprons, which provide limited protection to the arms and legs, consider using a set of lightweight, water-repellent coveralls. Several companies now sell disposable coveralls for around $4–$7 each. Although these lightweight coveralls won't protect someone from a thorough drenching, they do provide great splash protection for the entire body (including the lower arms and legs) and are comfortable enough to wear in the hot dryer area!

22. Can employees be disciplined for refusing to wear goggles and aprons when using dips and shampoos?

Occasionally, one staff member just refuses to follow the rules. When this happens, it undermines the effectiveness of the entire program. The hospital leadership must treat this situation like any other discipline problem. Keep a written record of every action taken. The following steps may be helpful:

• First, be sure the hospital's emphasis displays the **proper perspective**. Here are some examples of the wrong perspective: "You really should wear that stuff for your own good." "I'll get in trouble if OSHA comes in here and sees you not wearing your goggles and apron." Here are some examples of the correct perspective: "Janie, you have been trained in the safety principles rules of this practice, and I expect you to follow them." "Joe, I must assume that you still have questions about the safety rules of the practice since you're still not wearing the required protective devices." In the first examples, the leadership tried to enforce a rule without accepting responsibility; in the second examples, it is clear that employees are expected to follow the rules.

• Second, check **employee understanding** of the requirement. Provide additional training if necessary.

• Third, **specify** for the employee the parts of the program with which he or she is noncompliant. Most consultants advocate a verbal approach at this point, but be sure to keep a record of the conversation.

• Fourth, if the staff member continues to violate the safety rules, give them a written **letter of admonishment**. Many hospital leaders avoid this step because it takes time to do, but the use of a standard form or stock letter can make it easier. As a general rule, after this step the majority of employees adjust their behavior and no further steps are necessary.

• Fifth, follow the **disciplinary procedures** outlined in the hospital policy manual, but at this point many people advocate an administrative suspension without pay. Simply send them home for the rest of the day (or even 2 days) without pay.

• Finally, in the extremely rare circumstance that the employee refuses to follow the hospital rules, despite proper training and verbal or written reprimands, begin proceedings for **dismissal**. Most human resource managers and employment attorneys affirm that dismissal for failure to follow established safety procedures is legal, and, in most cases, the employee is not eligible for unemployment compensation. As always, this can vary by state or locality; if you have questions, be sure to contact a counselor familiar with your local situation.

23. Are there any safety restrictions on eating and drinking in the practice?

Yes. The potential for illness from ingestion of pathogens or harmful chemicals is present in most veterinary hospitals. Although some veterinarians joke that immunity only comes from exposure, OSHA is serious about rules against eating and drinking in hazardous areas. Several years ago, a veterinarian was fined for allowing employees to eat lunch on the treatment table. Although not specifically mentioned in OSHA standards, the treatment table is a potential contamination source.

Regulatory Matters 79

Consumption of food and beverages must be limited to areas free of toxic and biologically harmful substances. This rule also applies to *preparation* of foods and beverages. Many hospitals have a staff coffee and utensil area located in a lab storage area. Sometimes the cabinets above a coffee or food area contain hazardous chemicals or supplies. Hospital refrigerators are another area of concern: staff lunches, drinks, condiments, and snacks must be stored in an area free from biological or chemical hazards. Vaccines, drugs, and laboratory samples are potential contamination sources. It is acceptable to store patient food in a refrigerator with human food.

24. What is the difference between exhaust and ventilation?

Ventilation generally refers to bringing outside air inside to replace foul or contaminated air, but in some cases it means diluting high concentrations of fumes or vapors by mixing them with large volumes of air. Both replacement and dilution usually are accomplished by the building's heating, ventilation, and air conditioning (HVAC) system.

Exhaust generally refers to the removal of fumes or contaminated air at a specific location. Removal usually occurs by means of a dedicated exhaust fan *before* fumes accumulate to dangerous levels.

25. Is it important to record work-related accidents?

Yes. Every business should maintain a record of the details whenever an employee is injured or becomes ill because of their job. This is usually done by completing a Worker's Compensation Insurance Claim Form or similar accident report. An accident report must be prepared even if the business pays for the treatment and does not turn in the claim to the insurance company! It is permissible to use OSHA Form 101 as the accident report form, but it is not necessary to maintain two forms for the same purpose.

26. What are the parameters of "work-related" activities?

Generally, OSHA considers the employee's presence on the property as presumption of a work relationship even if they are not actively engaged in a work-related activity. For instance, if an employee is injured in a breakroom or restroom of the hospital, or slips and falls while picking up a paycheck but is not actually on duty, the injury still is considered work-related. The parking lot normally is not considered part of the workplace, unless the employee is in the parking lot performing a specific duty related to his or her job (e.g., cleaning the area or assisting with an animal). Even when state liability laws find the employer financially responsible, an accident that occurs during an employer-sponsored event, such as a picnic or outing, is not considered work-related for record-keeping purposes if attendance at the outing is voluntary.

When employees must travel outside the workplace to perform company business, they are considered to be on the job while traveling to the location, while performing off-site work, and while traveling back to the business, except if they are engaged in personal activities. For instance, if a receptionist making the bank deposit for the practice is involved in an automobile accident on the way to or from the bank—even in her privately owned vehicle—then any injuries she receives in the accident are considered work-related. Normally, commuting to or from work is not considered part of the work relationship for record-keeping purposes. However, if the employee runs errands for the business on the way to or from work, he or she is "on the job" as soon as the activity begins and is "off the job" when the activity ends and the normal route of travel is resumed.

Any injury that occurs while employees are performing tasks "in the interest of the company" should be recorded as occupationally related.

27. What is the OSHA Form 200?

OSHA mandates that each business with 11 or more employees (at anytime during the year) must maintain OSHA Form 200–Log of Occupational Injuries and Illnesses. If a business has more than one establishment, then a separate set of records must be maintained for each location, even though all employees are counted together in calculating the "11 or more" rule. Although the log may be maintained at an alternate location, an up-to-date copy (within 6 working days) must be present at the worksite at all times.

Any business that is required to maintain OSHA Form 200 must post the "Totals" section of the form on the employee bulletin board where notices are customarily posted. The summary for the previous year must be posted no later than February 1 of the current year and must remain posted until at least March 1. Do not post the entire form showing the names and job titles of injured employees; copy or cut the form where indicated and post only the totals section of the summary. Again—*only the last page containing the totals should be posted!*

28. Are animal bites and scratches considered recordable workplace accidents?

An occupational injury or illness is defined as any incident that occurs while an employee is working and meets one or more of the following conditions:
- the death of an employee
- diagnosis with an illness related to work activities

- an injury that results in loss of consciousness, medical treatment other than first aid, loss or restriction of work or motion, or transfer to another job.

Animal bites and scratches can quickly turn into problems that require medical treatment, even if first aid was performed at the time of the injury. For simplification, each practice should define exactly when an incident is considered reportable by the staff member. The local county animal control rules could be the guidelines. For example, all animal bites that break the skin and scratches that draw blood should be reported.

29. If a staff member sticks him/herself with a needle, is that considered a recordable accident?

Only if the needle has already been used on a patient, contains drugs or contaminants, or is no longer considered sterile.

30. How and when are accidents reported to OSHA?

Veterinary practices are not required to report individual incidents to OSHA or send accident reports or logs to OSHA unless the incident results in the death of an employee (incidents involving violence are included) or in the hospitalization of five or more employees from the same cause. The report should be made via telephone to the nearest OSHA office. Additionally, if the practice has received notice from OSHA that it has been selected to participate in an annual statistical analysis of workplace injuries or illnesses, then reporting guidelines will be provided with the notice.

31. What is the definition of a "needlestick injury"?

A stick with a dirty, used, or contaminated needle is an accident. A stick with a clean, sterile one usually is not considered an accident.

32. What should be done if someone does poke themselves with a needle?

If it was a clean needle, it's not really a problem; just wash the area with antiseptic.

If it contained a drug, read the precautions and information on the package insert and MSDS. Unless the drug is toxic or the person is allergic, there's probably not much to worry about. Use an antiseptic wash. When in doubt or if there is a chance the drug was injected (even a small amount), contact a poison control center and ask for advice.

If the needle was used for blood collection on animals, determine the likelihood of transmission of a zoonotic disease. If it is not probable, just antiseptic washing is indicated.

Always ask whether the injured employee wants to go to the doctor for a consultation and/or tetanus booster. If he or she wants to go, make the arrangements. If they refuse, no big deal; just note it.

An accident report should be completed for all needle stick injuries (except for sterile, unused needles), even if they seem minor at the time. Of course, not every incident is turned into the insurance company, but you do want to have a record of the situation if it turns into a problem later.

33. Must we have a separate x-ray monitoring badge for every staff member, even if they don't take a lot of x-rays?

OSHA requires that each person who is occupationally exposed to ionizing radiation be supplied with a personal dosimetry device if they can receive 25% of the allowable dose in any calendar quarter. This generally means that staff members must be provided with the badge and required to wear it if they participate in taking more than one or two x-rays a month. Staff members who do not participate in the exposure phase of the procedure are not required to have or use monitoring devices.

34. How often should x-ray badges be exchanged?

Monitoring badges should be exchanged based on the exposure. A monthly exchange is appropriate for practices that make many radiographs. A quarterly schedule is more appropriate for practices that take few radiographs or for those with consistently no record of exposure.

35. What protective equipment is required for the staff when taking radiographs?

Minimum protective equipment includes full-hand gloves and an apron that covers the torso with a rating of at least 0.5 mm of lead equivalency. Hand shields that cover just the top of the hands do *not* meet OSHA requirements for protective equipment. Mitts with a slit in the palm can be used if the animal's paw is pulled into the glove, but not if the staff member's hands or fingers stick out of the glove.

Thyroid shields and radiopaque glasses are recommended during fluoroscopy procedures, but are not required by OSHA.

36. What are the shielding requirements for the walls in an x-ray room?

Normally, the room where the x-ray machine is located must be shielded to prevent unintentional exposure to occupants of adjacent areas. In some cases, exterior walls or those that border unoccupied spaces do not require shielding because there is little chance of someone being on the other side of the wall when an x-ray is taken. If shielding is required, it should be a continuous barrier of $1/16$-inch lead (including doors) for fluoroscopic procedures or radiation therapy. However, in most cases, practices using only diagnostic x-ray machines can achieve adequate and effective shielding with two layers of sheet rock on the wall.

When newly installing diagnostic machines, a competent physicist should perform mathematical calculations of the proposed machine and room to determine the type and size of shielding required. This evaluation is very straightforward and reasonably priced. Check with the state health department or the radiology department of the local hospital to find a physicist who will do this work.

Whenever possible, the person operating the machine should stand behind a fixed or moveable shield. Newer shields are more affordable and allow a broader view than older ones. There even are shields that move on tracks on the ceiling so that no floor space is used! Contact your regular x-ray supplier, or Nuclear Associates at (516) 741-6360, for more information on shields.

37. Can the x-ray machine be located in the treatment area, or must it be placed in a separate room?

Unless state rules prohibit it, radiographic machines can be installed in the treatment room as long as the room is clear of people when radiographs are taken.

38. Can staff members under age 18 be allowed to take x-rays?

OSHA regulations do not specifically prevent minors from taking part in x-ray operations because there already is a federal law called the Fair Labor Standards Act that prohibits minors from performing specific dangerous tasks or activities. Exposure to occupational radiation is considered a dangerous task and therefore is prohibited for minors in the workplace.

39. Can the used fixer and developer be discarded in the sewer?

Normally the quantity, strength, and nature of the *developing solution* is of minimal concern for municipal waste treatment facilities, and it can be discharged into the sewer directly. Practices with septic systems should not dump this chemical into the drains because of possible damage to the microbe action that is the heart of the system.

The *fixer*, however, is another matter. Since fixer contains a heavy metal (silver), it should never be discharged directly into any sewer or septic system. Basically, there are two disposal methods available to the average practice: **filtration** of the fixer solution prior to disposal into the sewer, or **total removal** of the bulk chemical by a company in that business.

• Simple recovery units are available for automatic processors for less than $50. Recovery systems for manual developing operations also are available, but are slightly more time-consuming than the average practice is willing to endure. In any event, if this method is used, it is essential that the directions for the device be followed exactly and that the device be checked periodically and changed when necessary.

• Perhaps the best method for most practices is to contract with a licensed hazardous waste hauler to collect and properly dispose of the chemicals. Many x-ray suppliers will perform this service for their customers. There is usually a fee, but most practices feel it is worth the peace of mind.

40. Besides needles and sharps, what other items in a veterinary practice are considered hazardous medical waste?

• All waste from chemotherapy operations.

• Tissues from animals suspected to have a disease that can be transmitted to humans.

• Culture (bacterial, fungal, or viral) media with growth.

• Medical devices (e.g., blood tubes, IV bags and lines, and catheters) containing human pathogens or that have been used on an animal with a disease that can be transmitted to humans.

• Waste from animals infected with a disease contagious to humans (which can be transmitted by means of the waste).

• In some states (e.g., Florida), all materials used on nonhuman primates are considered hazardous medical waste.

41. Are pre-exposure rabies vaccinations required for staff members?

Although there is no direct requirement, OSHA's General Duty Clause does require employers to provide a workplace free from unnecessary dangers. In past situations involving other professions, when protection (such as vaccinations for hepatitis B) was available and the risk was found to be greater than in the average population (such as in human healthcare workers), OSHA has required the employer to provide the protection at no charge to the employee or to obtain the employee's written waiver of the vaccine.

In any case, it is necessary to inform the worker of the exact nature and degree of risk, as well as the everyday safety methods to use.

42. What emergency notification posters are required by OSHA?

Emergency telephone numbers, including fire, police, ambulance (or Emergency Medical Service), and emergency maintenance personnel should be assembled and prominently displayed near each telephone. Don't assume that everyone knows to dial 9-1-1 for an emergency. Since a few seconds could make the difference in an emergency, write down clear instructions and a "script" for the person to read.

43. Do I need an emergency plan?

OSHA's Employee Emergency Plans and Fire Prevention Plans Standard (1910.38) requires businesses to address all potential emergencies. The following are important components to consider when creating your emergency plan:

• **Emergency escape procedures**, including a floor plan or diagram that clearly shows the location of fire extinguishers, control valves, danger areas, and escape routes.

• Procedures to be followed by workers who remain to perform (or shut down) critical operations before they evacuate. This is usually not an issue in most veterinary practices since there are no critical operations that must be manned during an emergency.

• **Procedures to account for all employees** after emergency evacuation. Designate a central meeting place for everyone to assemble. This will make accounting for everyone fast and easy. Designate a person to take charge of the scene until emergency personnel arrive.

• **Rescue and medical duties** for those workers who are to perform them. This has limited application to the veterinary profession, unless the hospital is physically remote and professional medical or rescue personnel could be delayed in responding. In those cases, an adequate number of workers on each shift should be trained in basic first-aid for humans (such training also will comply with the Bloodborne Pathogens Standard). Training and certification are available through organizations like the American Red Cross or the local fire department.

• **The preferred means of reporting** fires and other emergencies. Appoint an individual to make the call. What happens if you must evacuate the building before the call can be made? Designate an alternate site, like a neighboring business or even a near-by phone booth. If you have a central alarm system, make sure everyone knows how to manually activate it.

• **The plan manager**, who can be contacted for further information or explanation of duties under the plan. Someone must be responsible for developing, updating, and explaining the details. Name this person in the plan. Make sure to keep the plan current.

44. Should I assign specific staff members to evacuate animals in an emergency?

There is considerable debate about the role of staff members in rescuing animals from the hospital in the event of a fire or natural disaster. OSHA does not require or prohibit staff members from participating in rescue duties; however, one major factor must be addressed—training. Just making evacuation part of an employee's job description is not enough. If staff members are required, encouraged, or allowed to participate in the rescue or organized evacuation of animals (or humans), then OSHA requires the business to provide adequate training on how to do the job safely.

If employees are expected to render first aid to people, then the business must comply with all the provisions of OSHA's Bloodborne Pathogens Standard. All things considered, most practices should leave the rescue duties to the professionals!

Note: when assigning duties for an emergency plan, make sure the staff member understands the task and is competent to execute it.

45. Are we required to post a floor plan for evacuations?

Although OSHA standards do not specifically require the posting of any evacuation diagrams, an evacuation diagram is a great start to your plan—after all, a picture is worth a thousand words! Use different colored inks or different symbols to mark the location of key components. For each fire hazard identified (e.g., oxygen tanks and hazardous chemicals), attach a simple control protocol for regular checks of the area and any special fire protection or suppression methods necessary. Mark the locations of smoke detectors and fire extinguishers, and indicate the last inspection date.

46. How many fire extinguishers are required for a veterinary hospital?

There must be enough fire extinguishers placed strategically throughout the hospital so that one is always less than 75 feet from any point in the building.

The rating and type of extinguisher depends on the function of the hospital and the chemicals that may be present. In general, most veterinary hospitals use dry chemical or carbon dioxide (CO_2)–type extinguishers, but check with your local fire marshal to be sure. Dry chemical extinguishers are known to be corrosive to electronic equipment, so ask the computer and laboratory equipment supplier for their advice also!

47. How often should fire extinguishers be inspected?

OSHA requires a program to ensure that fire extinguishers are inspected annually by a qualified technician. Most local fire departments perform this service automatically, but it's still the employer's responsibility to ensure it happens.

Maintain a record of the inspection. This can be done by placing a tag directly on the extinguisher, or by maintaining a log. Designate someone to visually check each extinguisher to ensure that it is still properly charged and hasn't been removed or damaged. Do this on a monthly basis! This monthly check should be annotated on the reverse side of the inspection tag. The date and person's initials are sufficient.

48. How many emergency exits are required in a veterinary hospital?
That depends on the layout of the hospital. In general, each area or section of the building (not necessarily each room) should have at least two emergency exits. Many hospitals have work areas that are located in basements or other isolated places. In those instances, ensure that the two means of egress will not be blocked by a fire or other emergency.

49. Is a window in the basement good enough for an emergency exit?
If the window is easily accessible—meaning you don't have to climb over furniture or materials to get to it. It must be no higher than 30 inches from the floor and meet the minimum size requirements for an exit or exit access (a corridor, hall, door, or other means that leads directly to an exit door), which are 28 inches wide and and 6 feet 8 inches high.

50. How should emergency exits be identified?
Exit doors must be marked with a sign bearing the word "EXIT" in plainly legible letters not less than 6 inches high and ¾ inch wide. Where the direction of travel to reach the nearest exit is not immediately apparent, a sign reading "EXIT" with an arrow indicating the direction must be posted.

Exits, signs, and egress routes must not be decorated or "hidden" so as to detract from their visibility. If an exit is not clearly visible, the route to it must be properly marked. Exit doors must not be locked or fastened in such a way as to prevent free escape from the inside of the building. In no circumstances should a dead bolt or lock requiring a key to exit from the inside be installed on an exit door!

51. I've heard that every door in the building must have a sign saying either "EXIT" or "NOT AN EXIT." Is this correct?
No, it's a myth. OSHA's requirement (and what makes the most sense) is to have the routes to exits, as well as the exits themselves, clearly marked. For instance, if a staff member is standing in the treatment room and cannot see a clearly marked exit, there should be signs over or on the doors leading to the exits. Note, however, that if a door can be mistaken for an exit (for instance an old exterior door that looks like a way out but is locked or blocked), then it must be clearly marked "NOT AN EXIT."

52. Are automatic emergency lights required in a veterinary hospital?

Power outages are common in some areas and rare in others. Nonetheless, they do happen. Veterinary hospitals must provide emergency lighting for areas where someone would have a difficult time finding an exit or may be involved in a hazardous situation when the power fails. Even for areas with exterior windows, it's important to assess the emergency lighting requirement; there isn't much light from a window when it's dark outside.

53. Are hand-held flashlights acceptable as emergency lights?

Not normally. Hand-held flashlights and ones that must be activated mechanically, however convenient, usually are not within reach during an unexpected power outage and are not appropriate emergency lights. Emergency lights must come on *automatically* when the flow of power is interrupted. If someone is involved in a procedure with an animal (e.g., bathing a dog, venipuncture of a patient, or a surgical/anesthetic procedure) when the power fails, only an automatic emergency lighting system allows them to safely complete or terminate the procedure.

54. Must we provide a first aid kit for employee or client use?

OSHA requires that a first aid kit be available when the workplace is not in "near proximity" to a hospital, infirmary, or clinic, or when normal Emergency Medical Systems (EMS) services are not available. If your city or county has an established EMS, then you should rely on their expertise in an emergency. In reply to several inquiries, OSHA has defined "near proximity" to mean "within 3–4 minutes of an accident involving suffocation, severe bleeding, or other life-threatening injuries . . . or within 15 minutes where a life-threatening accident or illness is unlikely."

Obviously, any situation can quickly become life threatening, but the key here is whether such a scenario is "reasonably expected." Access to emergency treatment within 15 minutes is the standard for almost every veterinary practice.

55. What if we don't have a hospital, physician, or EMS service in "near proximity"?

Then you *must* assemble a first aid kit. OSHA requires that a physician identified by the business owner determine the contents of the kit to meet the specific needs of that business.

Someone on each shift must be adequately trained to render the aid and properly use the supplies on a human patient. This mandates extensive training, usually through an agency like the Red Cross. Don't forget about the requirements of OSHA's Bloodborne Pathogens Standard. These very strict requirements do not *normally* apply to veterinary operations because there is no significant danger from a worker coming in contact with human blood or other potentially infectious materials from a human source. However, if the practice requires a person to be trained and available to render first aid to a human, then this person must be protected from the transmission of diseases from other humans. If an exposure control plan is required because of this standard, then compliance assistance from a safety professional is warranted.

56. If we are in "near proximity," does this mean I can't have a first aid kit in the practice?

Not at all. Most practices have found a happy medium with "self-aid" kits, in which common items like adhesive bandages and antiseptic ointment are available. If the injured person is not capable of self-aid, then the accident is serious enough to warrant treatment by a physician.

Mobile practices should follow the same rules as for a fixed installation. Have a self-aid kit available in each unit, but if the injury is more serious, use the cellular phone or two-way radio to summon EMS assistance.

57. Should I institute a policy that prohibits employees from rendering life-saving assistance to someone else in the event of an emergency?

These rules do not prevent a person from rendering assistance to anyone in need; they merely let each person decide when and how to place themselves in that position. The business can support an employee's decision to get additional training in human life–saving (such as Red Cross CPR classes), but if you make it a requirement, then you must provide a protection plan.

CONTROLLED SUBSTANCES

58. Are there any simple checklists for staying in compliance with the U.S. Drug Enforcement Agency (DEA)?

The many rules and regulations for DEA compliance can be overwhelming.

Checklist for Easing DEA Compliance

Registration
- Are all veterinarians who prescribe controlled substances, or cause them to be dispensed or administered on the premises, registered with the DEA?
- If the veterinarians administer or dispense controlled substances at more than one location (e.g., satellites), are they registered to each location with the DEA?

Table continued on next page.

Checklist for Easing DEA Compliance (Continued)

Registration *(cont.)*
- Is the registration current for each veterinarian (must be renewed every 3 years)?
- Is the current registration certificate maintained on the premises and available for inspection?
- Is the address on the registration current? (You must notify DEA of moves *prior* to the effective date of the move.)

Identification
- Are all drugs on the premises, regardless of their age or stage of use, identified as controlled substances?
- Are the most recent additions included, even if the package is not yet labeled?

Security
- Is there a substantially constructed, adequately secured container or safe available?
- Are stock levels kept to the minimum necessary for operations?
- Is an alarm system present when excess quantities must be maintained?
- Is the alarm system evaluated regularly?
- Is access to the storage area restricted to the absolute minimum number of employees?
- Are unopened bottles of any scheduled substance stored in the locked container?
- If working bottles are used, is there only one opened bottle out at any given time?
- Can you determine how many bottles, pills, etc. of each controlled substance you should have on hand at any given time?
- Can you identify shortages in a timely manner (at least monthly)?

Ordering
- Is DEA Form 222 available and access restricted to authorized personnel?
- Is DEA Form 222 used consecutively?
- Is DEA Form 222 maintained separate from all other accounting, financial, or hospital documents (e.g., its own folder)?
- Is the third copy of DEA Form 222 maintained on the premises for 2 years?
- Is the third copy of DEA Form 222 annotated when the drugs are received?
- Are telephone orders of schedule III, IV, or V drugs received and recorded by someone other than the person who placed the order?

Accountability
- Are schedule II drugs accounted for separately from other schedules?
- Are all scheduled drugs recorded to the patient level (records, receipts, etc.) when administered or dispensed?
- Are the logs orderly and readily retrievable for 2 years?
- If a computer program is used, has it been approved by the regional or state DEA office? (Some regional offices will not accept computer-generated logs.)

Table continued on next page.

Checklist for Easing DEA Compliance (Continued)

Accountability *(cont.)*
- Can you identify by patient and client name all animals who have received controlled substances from your hospital within the past 2 years?

Inventories
- Was the required initial inventory conducted and documented on the day you first engaged in controlled substance activity?
- Has the required biennial inventory been conducted and documented?
- Was the biennial inventory conducted on the required date (the anniversary of the initial inventory or May 1 of the odd years)?
- If the biennial inventory was not conducted on the prescribed date, has advanced written notification been made to the nearest DEA field office?
- Are periodic, unannounced spot-checks conducted to verify quantities on-hand?
- Are records of inventories maintained separately or in such a form that they are readily retrievable from other documents?
- Are records of inventories maintained for at least 2 years? (Some states, like Texas, have extended this time requirement, so please check.)

Shortages
- If there is a theft of controlled substances, has the nearest DEA field office been notified (DEA Form 106) in addition to the local police?
- If there is a significant unexplainable shortage, has the nearest DEA field office been notified (DEA Form 106) in addition to the local police?

Disposal
- Are drugs checked frequently for expiration?
- When drugs are expired, are schedule II and significant amounts of schedule III, IV, and V drugs sent to a "reverse distributor" for destruction?
- If local destruction is authorized (e.g., insignificant amounts of schedule III, IV, or V), are there witnesses to the destruction?
- Are balance-on-hand amounts adjusted only after proper destruction has occurred?
- Are records of destruction maintained for 2 years?

Prescription Writing
- Are prescription pads stored in a safe place to prevent misuse?
- Are DEA numbers *not* preprinted on the prescription pads, to reduce scams?
- Are all prescriptions for scheduled drugs noted in the patient's medical record?
- Are prescriptions for controlled substances written for the minimum quantity of the drug necessary?
- Are all telephone prescriptions (including refill authorizations) for schedule III, IV, and V drugs annotated in the patient's medical record?
- Are written prescriptions signed in ink by the authorized prescriber?
- Are prescriptions for scheduled substances re-evaluated after the first refill or every 6 months, whichever comes first?

LITIGATION CONCERNS

59. What is the possibility of being sued for malpractice?
The number of veterinary lawsuits increases each year, partially because we live in a litigious society, and partially because of the high emotional value of pets to their families.

60. How can I protect myself against lawsuits?
The best way is to improve communications.
• Actively listen when clients tell you their concerns about their pets.
• Recommend the best care for the pet. If the client chooses to do less, be clear about the possible consequences of that decision. Note the client's choice in the pet's file.
• Be clear, consistent, and courteous in all of your communications with clients. Communications include facial expressions and body language.
• Keep good medical records. This is your best defense should you need to go to court.
• Give estimates for all work, and have the client initial them.
• Keep clients up-to-date on changes in the estimate as the patient's care dictates.
• Use consent forms or note on the patient record if the client refuses pre-anesthesia lab work, diagnostic testing, or surgery.
• Always show compassion and care for the pet.

61. What is the best format for medical records?
Examine Section 1 of the AAHA Standards for Veterinary Hospitals. Their format is the standard for the profession.

We prefer a letter-size manila folder, with terminal digit, alphabet-based color coding (numbers require a cross-reference system that adds to the front desk work). We also use self-adhesive, horizontal dividers, so that each "top prong" holds only one animal. We like the "Welcome to Our Practice" form on the left side as the manila folder is opened, with client correspondence filed under it (this is the client information, with minimal patient description information).

On each self-adhesive prong on the right side, there is a pink (female) or blue (male) **patient data sheet**, with a **wellness checklist**, a **master problem list**, and a **medication refill tracking system** (sample forms are available in *Building The Successful Veterinary Practice: Programs & Procedures [Volume 2]* and in the Veterinary Practice Consultants Signature Series Monographs at www.v-p-c.com). *Note:* The patient data sheet can be used to screen household trends, which is particularly important when atypical morbidity and mortality is suspected.

Progress notes are on lined paper under the patient data sheet, with client and patient name at the bottom (prongs are at the top); for annotations, use the problem-oriented medical record format. The **Subjective-Objective-Assessment Plan** was made popular by the University of Illinois in the mid-1970s and has not changed much since then.

- After the date is the "client concern"—in the client's words.
- The "subjective" is just the history, and the "objective" is the findings of your own professional observations/exam.
- The "assessment" is what you tell the client you are treating the animal for; it's sometimes a tentative diagnosis. (A differential diagnosis seldom is used in real practice, since it is an academic pursuit and confusing to the staff for sequential contact.)
- The "plan" includes diagnostics, medications, procedures, and the expectation for the next contact (three Rs—recall, recheck, and/or remind).

62. Which are the best supplemental forms to add to a medical record?

Forms are not "added to a medical record." Forms are used to establish quality healthcare delivery habits and are dynamic instruments based on the healthcare required for the case.

The best supplemental forms are simply "break-and-stick" labels that affix directly to the progress notes, so that the chronological care of each patient stays organized and systematized (a picture is worth a thousand words). Pictures of dental arcades, eyes, body shape for dermatology, and even laboratory or surgical procedures can make annotation of medical records faster and easier.

The AVMA Directory has a simple hospitalization/authorization form (circa 1982), and there are sample forms available in *Building The Successful Veterinary Practice: Programs & Procedures (Volume 2)* and in the Signature Series Monographs at www.v-p-c.com.

63. How long do I need to keep medical records after the pet is gone?

Medical records should be held 3–7 years from last contact with the patient or client. Ask the state or province veterinary medical association for the specific ruling in your jurisdiction. When an animal dies or is euthanized, the final entry of the master problem list should show the date and cause of death. This is when the clock starts ticking.

Move the pink or blue patient data sheet with the master problem list to underneath the client welcome form. Remove the balance of the records for that animal from the active medical record file, and chronologically file them in storage for the required time.

5. RIGHTS OF THE EMPLOYED

ASSOCIATES' EVALUATION OF JOBS

1. Can a veterinarian who is not the owner manage a veterinary practice?

Absolutely! Today's veterinary practice is a totally different place for a nonowner veterinarian. Associate veterinarians often do not have the desire to be owners, but have the talent and desire to be the team leader. A nonowner manager can be the senior doctor in an absentee-owner scenario or the medical and administrative director for a corporate or cooperative practice.

2. How can I, as a nonowner, select the best position for myself?

There are several basic factors to consider: Have you selected the type of practice you want, including species, size, and specialties? Do you know where you want to live, how many hours you are willing to work, and what size community you want?

The **attitude of the workplace** is what makes survival possible; all other skills can be learned. Are they willing to give you time to learn?

If you want to seek a busy companion-animal practice, there should be over 400 transactions per doctor per month. A mixed-animal practice may be busy at 250 transactions, depending on the size of the area being covered.

Your key concern is **personal preference**. There are veterinary-specific employment brokerages (e.g., VetNetAmerica, VPC Brokerage) that will do "match making" between practices and potential candidates, negotiating salary, hours, and other expectations (the practice pays the finder's fee).

3. How do I know if I am being productive?

• Multiply an associate veterinarian's personal compensation by 5 to get the expected personal gross revenues production.

• A companion animal practice needs to produce in excess of $250 per square foot annually to be effectively utilizing the facility.

• A clinician with a balanced companion-animal schedule and case load should have pharmacy sales approximately equal to the diagnostic sales for the same period.

- When using linear scheduling for a companion-animal practice, a doctor can see about 20 patients a day; with high-density scheduling (two consultation rooms and a nurse per doctor), a doctor can see the same number of patients in a half day.

4. How can I evaluate the team around me?

In healthcare the best measurement is called **continuous quality improvement**. Each person is responsible for addressing his or her own sphere of influence and making tomorrow better than today, next week better than this week, next month better than this month.

Performance appraisals must be immediate and specific. This is not school; thus, a "C" average means an employee is doing poorly. Performance planning involves setting the learning goals for the next 90 days, including clear measurements of success, and then striving for that goal.

A team has a leader, knows how to score, and gets recognition from the coach when they do well. Does this happen when you are around? A team should be accorded respect, assigned individual responsibilities, and receive targeted and timely recognition (three Rs of staff development). Such a team will unquestioningly follow their leader(s) into the jaws of adversity.

DOCTOR CONTRACTS

5. How do I put a price on my time?

Your time is valuable! Answer these questions to calculate the value of your time:

1. What is your annual salary?
2. How many weeks a year do you work? (Don't include vacation weeks.)
3. How many hours a week do you work?
4. What is the annual cost of your fringe benefits (usually about one-third of annual salary)?
5. What are the overhead costs necessary to maintain your office (e.g., rent, equipment, heat, lighting, telephone)?
6. What are your annual expenses for travel, conventions, etc.?
7. What is the annual cost of salary and fringe benefits for your staff?
8. What are the annual overhead costs to maintain your staff?

Add your answers to questions 1 and 4–8.

Divide by your answer to question 2. The result is the **value of your time per week**.

Divide by your answer to question 3. The result is the **value of your time per hour**.

Divide by 60. This is the **value of your time per minute**. Multiply by 3 to determine the value of a 3-minute phone call. Multiply by 5 to establish the cost of a 5-minute interruption.

BENEFITS PACKAGES

6. Should part-time employees receive the same benefits as full-time employees?

With today's low unemployment, **job sharing** is far more advantageous than hiring staff part-time. If you hire them part-time the manager is accountable for their actions, but in a job-sharing situation the staff is accountable to each other for the outcomes! Your system should recognize the multiple-person equivalent with respective prorated benefits. Consider this: for every 20 hours of scheduled work, the employee accumulates 1 hour of paid absence time. This time can be taken in a minimum of 4-hour blocks with at least a 3-week notice to management.

In some medical plans, a part-time person is not eligible for health benefits. Consider giving a pet health insurance policy to each staff member as a holiday bonus. The practice can charge full rates, bill the insurance company, and receive an amount higher than the premium cost in return. Everyone wins!

7. Elaborate on the benefits of job sharing.

In some practices, each team has a number of job-share staff members, so that the group always is able to assign tasks, organize, and effectively cover the practice during open hours. These are the businesses that expect the staff to self-schedule and meet previously established goals.

8. What is a fair compensation for my staff?

Fair is in the eye of the beholder; equitable is a comparison between people and time. A fair and equitable compensation budget for a companion-animal practice is less than 43% of the gross income for **doctor clinical salaries** and **staff salaries** (W-2) combined. When there is no facility overhead, as with house-call or production ambulatory practices, the compensation budget can be increased since the overhead expenses are reduced.

Unskilled new-hire candidates should be started at about 50¢ more than a fast-food restaurant's hiring wage, given a raise of 50¢ at about 30 days of orientation when they are doing solo work, and then given another raise at 90 days post-hire when team fit, competencies, and personal strengths have been clearly identified.

Young associates should be started at about 19–20% of their projected annual revenues.

In a mature practice with over $1.5 million income a year, a **hospital administrator** (MBA or MHA level) deserves $50,000, and a **Certified Veterinary Practice Manager** (CVPM from the Veterinary Hospital Management Association) deserves $40,000, both with a productivity pay linked to production of excess net.

The **benefits package** is additional to the above percentages and compensation plan, and can be 3–4% of gross.

9. What is a good benefit package for a mature companion-animal practice?

The benefit package is not part of the W-2 taxable wage (compensation plan) and can be an additional 3 to 4% of gross. In the majority of veterinary practices, vacation/holiday pay, sick pay, workers' compensation insurance, medical insurance, and continuing education monies are a minimum employment benefit.

We are seeing vacation/holiday pay and sick pay rolled together into a **personal-days account** (e.g., employee accumulates 1 hour of personal time for every 20 hours scheduled work, time is taken in 4-hour blocks, and 75% must be used within the year it is earned). This benefit is for all employees, even the traditional part-timer, since more part-time jobs are being configured into job-share equivalents.

Association dues are a common benefit for practices that believe in supporting organized veterinary medicine. The payment of **disability insurance** for primary providers and **"first death" partner insurance** are two common benefits among veterinarians. **Pet health/medical insurance** (the nondiscount type) has become an interesting benefit for companion-animal practices, since the coverage actually produces net income for the practice. Some practices like to pay for **professional and DEA licensure** to ensure that the coverage stays current at all times.

A **retirement plan** is important for tenured staff. Young workers often do not realize the earning potential of early investment monies. It often is essential to bring a third party (financial planner) into the practice to explain this benefit.

6. ANCILLARY SERVICES

BOARDING

1. Is boarding a profitable expansion consideration?

Boarding has many competitors in the marketplace, but that doesn't mean it isn't profitable. If you look at the staff support requirement, one animal caretaker can handle about 33 animals per day. During nonholiday seasons, most boarding facilities drop to about 40% full, so 90 to 100 animal units appear to be the cost-effective point for a full-time kennel master. With a proper in-processing system, the boarding services should refer about 23% of their guests to the hospital for some from of healthcare.

A hospital costs about $140 per square foot to construct, and a boarding facility is about half of that if it is a stand-alone structure. If you expand your hospital at $140 a square foot, boarding will take far longer to recoup the expense of the expansion.

Bathing can be a very profitable side-light of the boarding operation, if you charge for a cleansing bath at every discharge. We call it a "cleansing bath" so the comb-out can be minimal.

2. What are the boarding space requirements?

Runs are preferred for dogs, and vertical condos are preferred for cats. A run is 3 feet × 5 feet minimum, 4 feet × 6 feet preferred; sizes are well described in the American Boarding Kennel Association (ABKA) publications; AAHA Design Starter Kit for veterinary hospitals; or Subchapter A, Title 9, Code of Federal Regulations. A cat-only facility can be easier, quieter, and more economical to fit into the practice space.

Ninety to 100 animal units are needed, so that the species mix will cause a variance in the space requirements. A play area may take up more space, but it is an attractive selling point, especially if behind a clean glass wall instead of bars or chain link.

3. What are alternatives to traditional boarding services?

Alternatives include:

• **Pet resort** with a resort manager and guest services, featuring people time in addition to automatically scheduled play time, often in the

"exploration zone" (playground for animals) rather than the yard or the back field.
- **Bed and breakfast** for cats and dogs, with historical tours or named suites. In some cases, VIP suites are indicated (8 feet × 6 feet or 8 feet × 8 feet), accessed by a 48-inch half door instead of bars, with beds, a towel bar with monogrammed towels, television, and windows to the outside.
- **Pet hotel**, hotel manager, spa services, and similar anthropomorphic terms, often associated with a boutique.
- A **"camp"** for field trial dog areas, including retrieving exercises, swimming sessions (stock tank), and socialization time.

GROOMING

4. Is grooming a profitable expansion consideration?

Grooming has many competitors in the marketplace, but unlike boarding, it is seldom a profitable pursuit in itself. Like boarding, with a proper wellness screening system, the grooming services should refer about 23% of their cases to the hospital for some form of healthcare.

A grooming operation should have 20-amp drying cages, usually stacked, as well as cage dryers, which can be an added expense. Many groomers want the practice to supply everything, and still they want 60% of their income, which causes most practices to lose money on grooming.

As mentioned in Question 1, bathing can be very profitable: if offered with boarding and ONLY summer cuts along with the cleansing bath at every discharge, the pieces meld together.

5. What are appropriate groomer compensation packages?

If the groomer is on practice salary, they can be converted to 40% commission, and the practice will fare okay. This applies only if the accountable grooming team is cutting eight or more animals per day. Most groomers who supply all their own supplies and equipment can be offered up to 50% of their fees, if they are cutting eight or more animals a day.

A groomer who only rents space must return to the practice at least what those same square feet would produce as a boarding facility for cats (cats are lower maintenance than dogs).

Caution: regardless of the groomer's status, the community will assume there is a practice linkage if they are in your facility. A failure to perform, substandard work, or sporadic hours become a reputation drain on the practice entity.

PET BOUTIQUES AND PHOTOGRAPHY

6. How does a boutique differ from a regular practice resale area?

A "regular resale area" in a veterinary practice is not really a resale area. It is a place where food and shampoo is stored in the public view so the staff does not have to "go in back and get it" when a client requests it. Seldom can a practice offer the product quantity and prices needed to become competitive in the community, especially in communities with large-format retailers or expanded feed stores. The word "boutique" infers that the resale area carries a special, exclusive line of merchandise. A boutique typically offers something the others do not, whether it be behavior management devices, animal picture key chains and jewelry, special species-specific stationery and scarves, or even a parasite prevention and control center. It adds a bit of unique flavor and "image" to traditional shelves and stacks.

A tenured staff member can be granted or sold a percentage of the boutique in most States and Provinces without concern for the practice act (this is a form of golden handcuffs for key staff). He or she gets a return on investment based on net income.

7. What makes a boutique successful?

The key to success varies by community. The boutique should carry something not readily available in the community, and at an appropriate price. The boutique must offer **the unusual** as if it were usual, or the usual as if it were special and unusual. Selection of **logo** and **imprinted merchandise** with the many breeds and species represented in the practice patient mix are essential if you do not want to alienate any single segment of the practice. The products must be of adequate quality and reasonable price that return trade is produced. A boutique will not survive on single-impulse–buy patrons.

8. What are special boutique services or products that have been successful elsewhere?

- A **drawing** for a free photographic portrait each month for patrons of the boutique. Pet photographers often provide free sittings because they know that if the photos are good, people will buy additional ones.
- **Seasonal promotions** linked with the practice promotions, including a drawing for a free pet health insurance policy for patrons of the previous 30 days during National Pet Month.
- A **nutritional center**, with signed veterinarian endorsement (posted sign) of the recommended diets for each stage of life.

- A **behavior management center**, with head collars, Kong toys, scat mats, and related behavior-modification aids.
- A **parasite prevention and control center**, with a built-in museum featuring a pre-positioned magnifying glass to see the vectors.
- **Linkage with the Humane Society**, so that the practice acts as an agent/outlet in adopting healthy puppies and kittens.

EXPANDED PATIENT SERVICES

9. List some examples of expanded patient services.
- Grading of patient teeth (per the four pictures on CET brochures) by nurses as a courtesy service during January and February.
- Explaining to owners of large-breed dogs the difference between early PEN-HIP and later OFA certification.
- Assisting clients in understanding the benefits of the wellness program on pet health insurance (over $200 of reimbursable care for less than $100 of premiums).
- Respite care (a hospice term) for seniors and other high-maintenance medical cases; larger "bedroom" units for animals that need medical care, while their owners take a break (vacation) from the care requirements.
- Fat farm (weight management) programs for chubby pets; inpatient program during the winter months, including a refeeding program (new diet habits), with lab numbers mailed or delivered to the family biweekly during the inpatient stay. Terminology is directly from human weight loss campaigns, so clients automatically understand the benefits.
- Economical and recurring behavior management appointments with the nursing staff, and telephone referral to behavior specialists as needed.
- Senior pet classes for the owners of animals entering their golden years (to teach about monitoring special needs at home).

10. What are other ancillary services that can be offered?
- Nurse home visits (protocols, procedures, and Pet Partner Program certification can be obtained from the Delta Society (1-800-869-6898).
- Day care for pets (day boarding).
- Support your local schools with Pets by Prescription, a pet library service, or classroom visitations; program details and outlines are available from the Delta Society (1-800-869-6898).
- Puppy classes, socialization and kindergarten, new-owner orientation, and similar introductory systems to teach the new owner or family about pet care. Affiliate with a dog trainer and/or sponsor space for the training classes.)

- Kitten carrier classes (the name is used to tell clients how a cat should be transported at all times), to orient clients about the most current care of cats.
- A practice lending library for animal books and videos, web site, and other client-education enhancements.
- Operation Pet I.D., with digital camera photos, name tags, microchips, tattoos, and "puppy passports" as anniversary gifts to clients, instead of reminders.

7. GROWING BEYOND ONE DOCTOR

FINDING AN ASSOCIATE

1. How do I find the best doctor for my practice staff?

Stay active in continuing education activities offered by your **local association** so that you know who is working in the area. Use the **veterinary distributors** that visit your practice as part of your search team. This is the most effective outreach program, since they know your practice and they also know who is looking. They can be very helpful in building contacts.

University **internship and externship programs** are a great source of doctors if you are willing to pay for them to be in your practice. The third-year externship program allows a budding clinician to "test your practice" while you get to see how they fit into your team.

The American Veterinary Medical Association **Job Bank** always has more jobs than doctors available, so you need to do more than just advertise a position to get appropriate applicants for your professional team. Advertising on the Internet, such as on the Veterinary Information Network, preselects for people who are computer literate—a strength in the new millennium.

When you start your search: look early, look regionally, and use every avenue available to get the word out on the benefits of joining your team.

2. What do I offer a new graduate?

First, this is a new generation of graduates: they want a personal life. This desire is not wrong. The days of the 60- to 80-hour practice week for doctors are over!

Second, benefit packages are important. Health insurance, continuing education, pre-tax support of dues, licensure, and related professional fees are minimum elements. Vacation, personal days, and flexible schedules, including recurring and scheduled 3-day weekends, are important benefits.

Third, the compensation should be productivity-based (since there are only so many doctor dollars in the budget), but many new doctors want a guaranteed base. This means that flexible budgeting and payroll programs are needed.

WORK AND PLAY WELL WITH OTHERS

3. How do I integrate others into the healthcare delivery team?

It is critical that you release control of a function only *after* you have trained someone to do the job and you can trust him or her to do it. Training should start as a directive process, and outcome expectations must be clear and consistent. Note that the practice's core values do not change from position to position; they are inviolate for everyone, even doctors. After the directive instruction, good leaders "persuade" the developing staff member(s) to try new procedures and demonstrate that they can be trusted. As the members try to apply the skills and knowledge to the new procedures, great leaders **coach without blame, mentor without appraisal**, and **use recognition** as the yardstick of developmental responsibility.

After directive training, persuasion, and coaching are completed, then and only then can delegation occur. *Outcomes are delegated, not processes.* Performance measures of success, established before the job is delegated, should include time lines. The delegation concept differs from single-doctor practice building because the process is released to the team member, who then has been delegated accountability of performance. After any delegation, the leader becomes the consultant to the staff member, but *never* takes the job back.

4. What are the key points to focus on initially when expanding the practice team?

Note that you must build the right model before you expand it.

• Build a management team that understands how to use a **program-based budget** (see Appendix B).

• Refocus attention from process to **outcome excellence**. Each management team member must understand "why" as well as "what," and the leader must develop the team's belief in the vision of the practice.

• Challenge the management team to become a **leadership team** by developing the practice vision in other staff members. Thus, the core values change from mere words to the working philosophy of the practice.

• Develop others on the practice staff to bond with clients, be patient advocates, and promote practice operational harmony.

EXPANDING THE TEAM

5. When do I expand my doctor staff?

Before you hire another veterinarian, expand your use of the paraprofessional staff; we call them **veterinary extenders**. Start scheduling rooms and tables, not doctors. Increase the use of outpatient nurses; implement high-density scheduling; and ensure that continuity of care issues are recorded in the medical records.

Not all practice owners can expand, due to demographics, the inability to release control (basic trust of others), or facility size. If any one of these three areas indicates poor potential, then focus on expanding your volume. Single-doctor practices start to reach peak performance at about 450 transactions per month. Most veterinary practices need to change from the doctor-centered habits that *built* the practice to team-centered programs that *grow* the practice (this usually requires about $500,000 gross income).

We suggest a staff ratio of four paraprofessionals to one doctor. In a single-doctor practice that leverages the staff and increases the staff-client contacts, the staff number can be double this traditional level and still have great performance.

6. I want to expand—when do I make that decision?

The reason for your decision to expand should be **client-centered**, not self-centered. Client demand must increase to make another doctor necessary for better client access. Conversely, client access should increase when a new doctor is added to the team. More surgery time, more appointments during surgery time, evening hours, greater weekend accessibility, and/or a wider scope of services will help justify hiring another doctor. Never hire a doctor to give yourself more time off and expect to grow net income.

At 450 transactions, the single-doctor approach with linear scheduling must change to prepare for another doctor. By using outpatient and inpatient nurses, nutritional counselors, dental hygiene specialists, parasite prevention and control assistants, and client relations specialists, the transaction rate can grow by 50% in a single-doctor practice (to 675 transactions).

At 600 transactions, one doctor with a good support team can still have a life. When the case load is 650 or higher, most practices will require another doctor.

7. How can I afford to expand the practice team?

A team should be worth every penny they cost and more. For the cost of a few dollars per hour, hundreds of dollars an hour can be generated—if you have trained to a level of trust.

The recovered patient program and recovered client program can produce an additional $150,000 per year with little change in overhead. Implementation involves recovering one lost client or patient every day, by using the three Rs: recall, recheck, remind. Look to improving efficiencies before expanding staff.

A **nutritional counselor** can effect 30 to 60 additional clinic visits a month. Your practice must have the discipline to share the rewards with the outpatient staff that will be needed to keep this wellness outreach program operational in the client's mind.

A **dental hygiene specialist** can effect 20 to 30 dentistries a month, especially in grades one and two dental hygiene levels. These are easier dentals, usually not requiring doctor involvement for extraction. Your practice must provide the training and share the rewards with the nursing staff to build a dental program.

Nursing telephone outreach can greatly increase client return rate. Under-staffing, compounded with low wages, often makes this task a last priority instead of a primary responsibility of a caring veterinary healthcare team. Give the staff adequate time to perform this critical bonding function.

8. How do I build from within?

There must be a progression of development and responsibility within any healthcare team, and veterinary medicine is no different. People need to know how they can advance. In some positions, like animal caretaker, the title and money may grow with the individual's tenure, but the core job does not greatly change. Additional duties can be added to allow greater practice worth, but caretakers primarily feed, scoop poop, and bathe animals.

Continuing education can develop skills and knowledge to allows other team members to develop to a higher level of performance. The Internet distance learning programs for veterinary technicians, local courses in client relations (e.g., banks, hospitals) and the Certified Veterinary Hospital Manager program offered by the Veterinary Hospital Managers Association (VHMA) are but a few investments a practice can make to develop its staff from within.

A skilled practice consulting team can assist in developing accountability and can provide the training to make the transition possible. See the Veterinary Consultant Network survey data from 45 national consultants for guidance on selecting a consultant (www.v-p-c.com).

9. How do I start the process of moving my practice to the "next level"?

When you walk through the front door of your practice, what is the atmosphere that you have created? Is there an open friendliness, or is there a fear of failure that prevents change? **Continuous quality improvement** must be a practice expectation.

Establish quarterly instead of annual performance planning. **Quarterly appraisals** allow you to fix problems while they are small and keep everyone focused on their goals.

The quarterly performance plan is a **joint effort**. Planning does not stop until the measure of outcome(s) and operational limits are established between the mentor and the staff member. The plan should include a time line and milestones for checkpoints and progress recognition. Your doctors' fear of lack of control is just as detrimental as the fear of failure. It derails the delegation process and delays the development of the healthcare delivery team. Always be honest with yourself about this!

10. Should we incorporate our practice/business?

One of the reasons often cited for incorporating a practice is the liability shield afforded a company's owners. Legally, a corporation is considered a "person" with its own identity, separate from the "identity" of the individual owners of the corporation. Theoretically that means that should the company be sued and lose, only the corporation—not the individuals who own the corporation—would be responsible for paying court-ordered damages.

Life being what it is, however, theory and practice often are two different animals. Such is the case with corporations and very small businesses. The reason: if you incorporate as a **one-person operation** and later do something that exposes you to legal liability, both the negligent person (e.g., you) *and* the corporation are liable. *You cannot excuse your own misconduct merely by incorporating.*

Similarly, incorporating a one-person or very small practice seldom protects the owner(s) from liability should the corporation default on a loan or lease. Banks, landlords, and others often require personal guarantees on loans and leases. If you make such a guarantee, then the corporate form of business will have no effect on your personal liability.

The situation is different, however, if you have staff members. If an employee is making a delivery for you and injures someone in a car accident, he could be held personally liable to the victim, as could the corporation through a legal doctrine called **vicarious liability**. However, because the corporation is a separate entity from the shareholders (owners), their personal assets would be protected.

Even if you have employees, you could inadvertently leave yourself liable for damages through something known as the **alter ego doctrine**, which is part of a legal remedy known as "piercing the corporate veil." If your corporation is a general corporation rather than a close corporation, you must treat that corporation as a separate entity in all of its formal and legal respects. If you don't, both you and the corporation could be successfully sued by an injured party on the grounds that the corporation is no more than the "alter ego" of the owner. The Limited Liability Corporation (LLC) or Limited Liability Partnership (LLP) usually has greater taxation issues than a Sub-S, and a C Corp usually has a better structure for retirement investments. Local legal advice and estate planning information will be needed to research the various tax consequences and succession planning issues.

11. What other issues besides liability should be considered before deciding to incorporate?

The corporate structure may require you to observe certain **legal formalities** regarding the way you run your business, and may expose you to **taxes or annual fees** that do not have to be paid if the business is a sole proprietorship or partnership. It usually is smart to "exteriorize" the building and land into a family estate with multiple owners, so they are not part of the estate upon an untimely demise.

Some small practices do benefit from incorporating. For example, the business' **image** may be enhanced. Depending on circumstances, incorporation may have **tax benefits** as well. The bottom line: consult with both your attorney and your accountant, and get all the facts you need to make the right decision for your business.

FEES AND VALUING HEALTHCARE

12. How do I set reasonable fees?

The traditional method is to attend a local Veterinary Medical Association meeting and swap tall stories with other practitioners. This has nothing to do with profit or practice, it is just what we do!

Know where your costs lie. A mature companion-animal practice should have a P & L monthly overhead less than 50% (without rent, doctor monies, or return on investment). If overhead is on target, prices are reasonable. A mixed practice's fees can be plus or minus 15% of the companion-animal practice's, depending on client and patient mix. As long as the net is better this year than last year, the practice is evolving in the right direction.

Know what each procedure costs you, including all overhead factors. You can then determine the net you want to receive on that procedure, and adjust your prices accordingly.

13. How do I know when my prices are exceeding the community comfort zone?

In most cases, as a result of negative customer feedback, the doctor will curtail fees before the whole community is aware. As long as your practice is within 10% of the top of the marketplace, quality and value can make the practice a bargain.

Value comes with client education; in the absence of knowledge, clients make decisions based on price. The nursing staff can educate, but the pride shown by the staff when presenting the invoice or healthcare plan costs will be perceived as quality. In healthcare, **high pride = high quality; indifference = mediocrity.**

8. CLIENT/CUSTOMER SERVICES (SMART MARKETING)

CLIENT VERSUS CUSTOMER

1. What is the difference between a client and a customer?

Customers = buyer beware! Clients have a social contract with a healthcare provider. The relationship between a veterinary healthcare provider and the pet owner is one in which the provider will speak for the animal's best interests. The client then has the right to accept or waive the animal's rights to that level of care.

Clients often come to a veterinary practice with apprehension and fear. They do not know what is needed or how much it will cost. Customers go shopping with a song in their hearts and the knowledge that they can walk away if the "deal" is not the best for them.

Customers expect to be pampered and served by the establishment, while clients often are given tasks and directions by a healthcare provider.

Clients expect quality care for their animals at an equitable price. This social contract is inviolate, and if the provider violates the contract, trust is lost and the bond is broken. In shopping, clients accept the responsibility for finding the best quality bargain at the cost they want to pay.

LONGER HOURS OR BETTER SCHEDULING

2. When should I consider expanded hours?

The hours your practice is open should depend on your client community and the **client demand**—not your preference to sleep in or go home early. Drop-off privileges for established clients may preclude the need to expand hours. This option requires a well-trained nursing staff for admission screening.

A "bedroom community" in a metroplex may not need morning or midday appointment hours at all. Accommodating these clients may mean accepting animals the night before during the standard outpatient hours (e.g., 4 PM to 9 PM). A rural community may not need expanded hours since most families have flexible farm or ranch schedules.

3. I am currently doing "9 to 5" veterinary hours, and the late-in-the-day appointments are filling 2 weeks in advance. Do I need to expand hours?

Whenever your clients can't get an appointment the same week, your client access is too limited. Clients want to see you within 24 hours of their call, so make it happen! Saturday crowds and late-in-the-day appointments are indicators of two-income families: they are the real reason to have evening hours. As these clients are seen, they can be given the value-added pitch—"You are now qualified for the preferred client drop-off privileges."

If you are telling clients they cannot come in this week, for any reason, you are negatively affecting your word-of-mouth referrals. This will reduce your new clients and limit the practice's growth.

Hire a doctor who "hates mornings" and expect him or her to only work noon to 9 PM. Such a schedule often is a benefit to everyone concerned. This doctor comes to work ready to do 3 hours of spay and neuters or other inpatient/call-back work, then outpatient appointments from 4 PM to close. He or she is fresh and highly productive at a time when others' energy is flagging, so everyone wins!

PRICE SHOPPERS

4. How do I best serve the price shopper?

"Shoot and scoot" vaccination clinics and "pay and spay" population control clinics will always be out there; let them have these price shoppers!

Price is relative. If the client's expectations are exceeded, then the cost of the service was reasonable. If the expectations are not met or exceeded, the client will perceive that too much was paid.

Around 30% of a companion-animal practice's clients provide approximately 80% of the annual income. If you are looking to serve a client group, profile the top 30% of clients (regular customers, those who pay on time, etc.) in your practice, and make them your concern!

5. Does persistence sell in healthcare delivery?

Yes! When a phone shopper contacts your practice, send **product literature** and/or a **practice brochure** within a day or two. If a week or more goes by without a visit or call from the prospect, take action! Doing nothing is a big mistake.

Potential clients who request literature or information often have a genuine interest in finding a quality healthcare practice, but they may not need your services immediately. Thus, they look over what you send, but put it aside for possible followup in the future. Months later, their priorities shift. Suddenly, the service or product they were thinking about purchasing "sometime" becomes what they need *now*. However, that first piece of literature you sent may be filed, misfiled, buried at the bottom of a stack of things to do, or even tossed out during a kitchen table cleanup campaign.

Position your practice to win those delayed sales by **following up regularly** for at least 6 months with newsletters or reminders. Make your initial followups once every month for 6 months if the prospect seemed genuinely interested. After that, followup with your quarterly newsletter. Newsletters or health alerts don't have to be elaborate or costly; even a postcard with a reminder to check your web site for new information is beneficial. Notices of special programs are good ways to keep in touch and keep your name and practice scope fresh in potential clients' minds.

6. What is the most effective coupon/discount technique?

In most practices, there is less than 20% true net in any average client transaction, so why give away any of this money? The best way to take advantage of coupons is to offer a special promotion. Look at **expanding client and patient access**, for example by offering "two-fur-one" (misspelling intentional) fecals for multi-pet households. This way, stools from two animals will be brought into the practice, often revealing other pets that require services or are unknown.

Seniors tend to expect discounts. As more of the American citizenry moves into the senior demographic, you will have more clients expecting discounts. Some practices add extra time to the standard appointment during midday and offer this as a "discount period." Midday typically is slow, and retired persons prefer to drive between rush-hour crunch times, so both practice and client can win!

MAKING THE FRONT DOOR SWING

7. What causes a reduced client flow?

Usually, something happened to adversely affect the client's image of the practice, e.g., major fee increases, poor client relations by doctor or front staff, or over-booking and turning away clients. This changed image is very difficult to correct, since word-of-mouth is working against you.

In some cases, a new "volume practice" has opened its doors and created a media blitz about economical vaccinations. Your practice still bundles quotables with a consultation and appears out-of-line with the competition.

If your practice has an 80% or better appointment log fill rate, the good news is that you are busy. The bad news is that you are limiting client access, and some are going elsewhere.

In some communities, the phrase "Appointment Required" litters the yellow pages and phone greetings. The message "Walk-ins Welcome," which conveys accessibility and convenience, causes a 25% increase in new client access.

8. When we drastically increased our prices last year, we celebrated the immediate increase in income. Now we see the ill effect in return trade—a 30% drop in repeat visits. What can we do?

First, quit kicking yourself—it does no good.

Second, commit to a **media blitz** that highlights "new access" services to established clients: day drop-off, economical vaccination visits, preferred client programs, "two-fur-one" programs, walk-ins welcome, etc. You must precede the media blitz and new **client information/education programs** with **staff refocus** and promotion education.

Third, make a **total commitment** to the new changes. It takes 7 to 10 years to reverse a bad community reputation in healthcare delivery.

9. We would like to do walk-ins, but they disrupt our scheduling. What can we do?

Often said in jest but founded in truth: "The day would have been great except for those clients." This attitude will kill a practice. The client is why we are in this business of veterinary healthcare delivery!

If high-density scheduling is embraced (two rooms to one doctor, scheduled out-of-sync [last 10 minutes and first 10 minutes overlap in the two rooms]), then one room is scheduled in the traditional manner, and the second room can be used for walk-ins, filling the seam positions. In a multi-doctor practice, the inpatient doctor team takes all walk-ins via an empty room (one reason why hospitals are designed with an odd number of consultation rooms). If a walk-in consultation room is not available, always offer two "yes" options: admit for daycare and waive the day inpatient fee (you would not have gotten it on outpatient), or tell the client when a time is available later in the day.

Never allow a walk-in client to hear or feel that they were a "work-in" client. Such communication of aggravation and/or disdain violates the social contract of healthcare delivery.

10. What is this "new social contract" of healthcare delivery?

It's not new; it goes back to the original covenant to Noah: "Tend to the animals of this land, keep them healthy, and allow them to populate the lands." The contract has four parts, starting with the traditional Greek medical premise, "First, do no harm!" The other parts are: do only what is needed; restore wellness in the patient; and assign fair and appropriate remuneration.

The social contract is an unspoken commitment made by opening the doors of a hospital. It is not optional; it is a common expectation—of the client, the staff, the local regulatory agencies, and responsible doctors.

11. How can we expand clinic hours without killing ourselves?

In one-doctor practices, you cannot do this easily. It requires additional nursing staff used as veterinary extenders, strategically planned appointments, scheduling the consultation rooms rather than the doctor, increasing drop-offs, and, possibly, sharing client support with other practices (called a "rotary" in Europe).

In multi-doctor practices, consider 2-week schedules instead of the traditional one. Again, schedule the rooms, not the doctors. Plan a doctor's schedule with two days on, one off, three days on, one off, four days on, then three days off. Start the second doctor on the same schedule, but one week out-of-sync. Consider Tuesday and Thursday evening hours, with a delayed late-morning arrival for the evening doctor.

When hiring a single (no significant other) doctor, a one-week schedule is possible if he or she hates mornings. Schedule work 11 AM to 8 PM on Tuesdays and Thursdays, 8 AM to 7 PM on Fridays, and 8 AM to 3 PM on Saturdays. This arrangement allows Saturday afternoon to Tuesday late morning off, as well as all day Wednesday and Thursday morning. The best part of this schedule is that *you* will have Friday, Saturday, and Sunday off every week . . . smile when you think about this!

12. Any other tips on scheduling?

When the doctor schedules are developed 6 weeks in advance, the staff has the opportunity to plan their respective schedules to match, giving themselves extended days off on a recurring basis. Note that it is not unusual to give an incentive pay differential of 75¢ per hour to staff working after 6 PM or on weekends.

WELLNESS PROCEDURES

13. Should my practice be selling dog food?

First, in quality veterinary healthcare we do not sell pet food; we sell **peace of mind**.

Second, there is no animal alive that can survive without some form of nutritional intake. The veterinary practice can balance life needs with nutritional intake parameters and extend the lives—as well as the quality of life—of their patients. You're selling the **benefits of nutrition** rather than the food per se, and offering clients something they can do for the members of their family with fur, fins, or feathers. The most rewarding aspect for clients is watching their pets thrive on a premium, balanced diet.

Nutritional counseling is the purview of the nursing staff. They are the nutritional advisors and can share the value of quality food. They can make 25–40% net, which is valuable to the practice. The key issue is benefits: cat food offers better-smelling litter boxes; dog food offers smaller, firmer stools; balanced, quality diets offer longer lives, better hair coats, and higher digestibility (fewer internal complications).

14. How do I sell more fecal tests to my clients?

First, in quality veterinary healthcare we do not sell fecal tests; we sell **peace of mind**.

Second, the Centers for Disease Control in Atlanta has stated that strategic deworming is essential in controlling larval migrans, a condition affecting over 15 million Americans in 1999. Your clients deserve to know about these threats to their family.

Third, many internal parasites (e.g., Giardia) are not prevented with the current combined heartworm medications, and must be screened for using special procedures (e.g., zinc sulfate float, direct smears).

Note that the staff should conduct parasite prevention and control counseling *after* the doctor's consultation and prioritization of healthcare, *not before*. The client's presenting concern must be addressed first; only then will he or she listen to your supplemental wellness healthcare messages.

15. How do I sell pain management?

First, in quality veterinary healthcare we do not sell pain management . . . (Can you finish the sentence? See Questions 13 and 14.)

Clients expect pain medication. If they ever had a potentially painful hospital procedure, pain management was prescribed and administered—it was not an option.

Initiate a **pain scoring system** within the practice team so that any trained nurse can track pain levels in patients. Pain scoring programs are available from the Veterinary Compendium, Veterinary Emergency and Critical Care Society (VECCS), and Signature Series Monographs (at web site www.v-p-c.com).

Consider including the pain injection in the bundle for every surgery, just as anesthesia is included, and then offer an upgrade to a patch. Here is a possible narrative:

> *"Pain control is essential with this procedure, so we have included a 12- to 24-hour pain control injection in the procedure price. But for only an additional $22.50, we can use a patch which extends the pain management for 3 to 5 days. Which do you prefer today?"*

16. How do I sell preanesthetic blood screening?

What do we sell in quality veterinary healthcare? (See Questions 13 and 14.)

Answer the following question truthfully: "For which animal, which species, which sex, what age, which breed is it *always* safe to do general anesthesia without blood screening?" Accept the current standard that the minimum preanesthetic blood screening includes packed cell volume (PVC), total protein (TP), and blood urea nitrogen (BUN) and include it in the bundle price as you do anesthesia for surgery. More tests may be necessary in older or distressed animals.

Consider using this narrative:

> *"We need to assess what is happening inside the body before anesthesia, so we have included the minimum level of tests in the procedure price (less than $10). However, we would prefer to do a full blood panel today. With a full panel screening the basic 12 (14) blood chemistries, if anything goes wrong in the next year, we will have the annual baseline to compare to and can act quicker. Which would you prefer today?"*

17. How do I sell intravenous fluids with surgery?

By now, you know the first part of the answer to this question.

As for the second part, clients expect fluids during surgery. If they ever had surgery, it was not an option. The State of Nevada Veterinary Board posed this question to VECCS, and they jointly determined that 80% of all surgeries require fluids during the procedure. A state board policy to this effect has been published.

We promote IV TKO (to keep open) slow drip with surgeries, so that an open IV is ready for rapid treatment should anesthetic misadventures occur. If this is done with an isotonic solution and single IV set, then connected to the catheter with an extension tube in case of blood back-flow, one bag of fluids can be used for 5 to 8 surgeries, and you can keep the IV TKO price to less than $10.

Consider this narrative:

"We need to assess what is happening inside the body before anesthesia, so we have included PCV, to tell us if there are enough red blood cells to carry oxygen and nutrients; TP, to tell us about the dehydration level and how much fluid therapy is needed during the procedure; and BUN, to tell us what the kidney can detoxify from chemicals in the body, in the procedure price. This is the minimum level of tests and costs less than $10, but we would prefer to do a full blood panel today. With a full panel, screening the basic 12 (14) blood chemistries, if anything goes wrong in the next year, we will have the annual baseline to compare to and can act quicker. Which would you prefer today?"

18. How do I pay for a new piece of diagnostic equipment?

The piece of equipment must earn its way, which means it must be used on a recurring basis. In today's competitive delivery market, it is smarter to do more procedures at lower prices than fewer at higher prices.

If you are looking at one of the new thoracic wall cardiac monitors (e.g., Biolog, Heska, PAM), then you must start doing more cardiac evaluations. If a cardiac evaluation is added to every Annual Lifecycle Consultation at less than $5, the monitor will pay for itself within 6 months and become a net-net benefit to the practice and patient.

If you are looking at a CO_2 laser surgery unit, accept the fact that declawing is a commodity item and cannot be priced as laser surgery. Reposition your practice to do laser surgery declaws on cats so that clients know the benefits in terms they understand, such as: (1) it allows a faster and easier anesthesia time, (2) pain *always* is less, and, most importantly (3) their kitty can go home the same day!

19. What makes a healthcare program appealing?

• Doing the unusual as if it were the usual, or the usual as if it were unusual. Thumbing the practice's nose at traditional paradigms and biases.

• Confronting and redefining an emerging community issue in such a way that colleagues and competitors alike remember it years later.

• Moving at record speeds and strategically responding to an emerging need, internal or external.

• Building dynamic and stimulating bonds with clients and staff.

• Measuring success in terms of caring, compassion, "gee whiz" comments, and revolutionary impact.

It starts with *you!* It is cemented by *you!* And most importantly, it embraces *your* core values and practice image!

MARKETING PERSPECTIVES

20. In a mature practice, what should my new-client rate be?

New clients should comprise 10% of all transactions each month. When numbers get down to 5%, the practice is dying in most communities. When they exceed 15%, the team generally is not bringing the clients/patients back often enough. Once clients are cycling (after 12 to 24 months), about 30 new clients a month are expected per FTE doctor in mature communities and 40 per FTE doctor in an expanding community (see Chapter 1 for FTE discussion).

It is not enough to have an attractive building, good equipment, and medical expertise. You have to figure out how to sell what you've got if you're going to succeed in practice. The following 10 questions and answers will help you think through what you're doing, avoid common mistakes, and make better marketing choices for growing your practice.

21. What's the single most important decision I can make for my practice?

Location, location, location. A well-located practice has a hard time failing. A good location means:

- The sign and building are visible to passing traffic.
- The building is attractive and inviting.
- It's easy to get to from the road.
- There's sufficient parking.
- The space is affordable.

In the case of specialty referral practices, all of the above are null and void. All clients come by way of maps provided by the practice's real clients—the practices that refer to the specialty practice.

22. How much money should I be spending on Yellow Pages advertising?

After location, a Yellow Pages listing(s) is your next most important marketing decision. Carefully select the book(s) you'll be in to target the clients you want. Keep expenses under control by choice of ad size and colors. Your phone listing should be visually attractive and stand out from the others, which does not necessarily mean it should be larger. Rather, differentiate yourself by highlighting your location (possibly include a map) to help convenience-oriented pet owners select your practice, and by advertising any special services you provide, such as handling of exotics, alternative medicine, boarding, grooming, and prescription food. These techniques will build traffic for your hospital.

23. Are "on-hold" phone messages a good idea?

Yes! The worst thing you can do is have nothing playing when people are on hold. Silence while holding makes the wait seem longer, and callers may think they've been disconnected. Short, informational, on-hold messages make sense. You can remind pet owners of things they should be doing for their pets, like heartworm checks, dental cleanings, and special diets. Tell clients about new products and services your practice provides.

Do not use on-hold time for sales messages. The client may think he or she has been placed into phone limbo just to hear the advertisements. Rather, think of the short phone messages as an audio newsletter for your practice.

24. What's an easy, effective marketing activity for my practice?

Use office displays that tie in with seasonal issues. For instance, when the weather starts to get colder, list the signs of arthritis in pets to help pet owners recognize symptoms. Tell pet owners what to look for, and let them know that you can help their pet—this is always a good idea! The more pet owners know, the more they'll do for their pets. Amplify the impact of your office's display by mailing information about new arthritis treatments to clients.

Always educate your staff about the promotions first, and ask for their help. Since they have the first contact with the client, they need to be knowledgeable—and they usually have great ideas.

25. What do I say when the local Little League, High School Yearbook Committee, or other group comes knocking on my door for donations?

Always ask yourself, "Does this make sense for my practice?" This question doesn't mean you should not support your community. These advertisement donations are just that: community charity.

Ask yourself what is most important to you. If you think it would be smarter to limit your donations to pet-related causes, then do just that. For instance, you and your staff could organize a dog wash and donate the proceeds to the local animal shelter. This would bring people to your hospital, earn goodwill, and help pets. It's the kind of donation that does you good while doing good.

If you believe in the youth of your community and want to help them, then the decision is not a management concern: the donation is a community service and a personal commitment. If it feels good, and you like the feeling of helping the group, then just do it!

26. Do I have to be open 24 hours to be competitive?

No. But you do have to be open at smart hours. Ask yourself, "What are the busiest days of the week at my hospital?" "What are the busiest times each day?" "What appointment hours do clients ask for that we don't provide?"

You may find that you can work fewer hours if you match the hours you are open to those that are best for your clients. For instance, you may be able to close Fridays at noon if you'll work until 3 PM on Saturdays. You may be able to close all day on Wednesdays if you provide early drop-offs and late pick-ups on the other days of the week.

27. Do I need a lot of staff to provide good client services?

No. You need a few well-trained, competent, outgoing people to make a good impression. Quality wins over quantity every time. When a practice is understaffed or there is a "disposable staff" attitude, the lack of quantity often hurts quality. Smart scheduling and training can make your practice run smoothly with fewer people, especially if they're the right people.

Note that when a doctor is doing nursing work (e.g., IV systems, anesthesia induction, x-ray position, laboratory procedures, nail trims), you have an understaffed hospital or too many doctors.

28. How can we use coupons to improve our marketing?

Coupons do not produce net. Most mature veterinary practices, after deduction of rent, ROI, and adequate clinical salary, have a less than 15% net income. Therefore, by simple math, using a 10% discount coupon requires three times the business just to break even. At 20%, like some of the "big-promise couponers" are offering, the practice will never make money on the coupon trade.

Coupons are a form of name recognition, and, if used strategically, they can help build an awareness of a new practice during the first 18 to 24 months of operation. However, to go beyond awareness you must have a staff trained to bring in repeat visits after the first coupon use. Some practices have successfully used a "come get to know us" coupon system to make the front door swing, but the staff was well trained in establishing the expectation for the next visit and getting the client to come back.

People who "follow the coupon" are not bonded to their veterinary practice and, in most cases, will not bond to a new practice. Bonded clients visit their preferred veterinarian 3 to 6 times a year (as established by the practice's expectations), while coupon clients most often "go with the flow."

29. How can we use the "Welcome Wagon" most effectively?

The use of a Welcome Wagon or other new-resident visitation agency is seldom a client-producing event, *unless* the visitation agent is a bonded client of your practice. Most communities now have multiple veterinary practices, and 60% of new residents look first at the location. The second thing they do is ask a neighbor for a recommendation (in good practices, 60% of new clients come from word of mouth). Thus, a visitation agent who makes a **personal recommendation**, rather than just leaving "paper," makes a difference.

Some Welcome Wagon programs require that a premium or discount be offered. After deduction of rent, ROI, and adequate clinical salary, most practices have less than 15% net income. Therefore, any "free" premium offer or discount coupon requires many more times the business than can be generated by the visitation program.

Welcome Wagon and other visitation programs can provide **name recognition**. If used strategically, with a staff trained to affect repeat visits after the first coupon use, they can help build an awareness of a new practice during the first 18 to 24 months of operation.

30. Is a newsletter a good idea for my practice?

In general, yes. Since it takes at least five exposures to get a client "yes" when they *know* their pet needs a procedure or service, and over a dozen when they *don't know* of the need, a newsletter can provide some of these exposures.

Newsletters are not "calls to action," and if they are expected to create business by themselves, they usually are ineffective. If the newsletter is attractive, inviting, interesting, and fun to read, it can be an excellent medium to stay in touch with your clients. Quarterly newsletters usually work best. They allow you to address seasonal issues, and they are less work and more cost-effective than monthly newsletters. Newsletters also are a good vehicle to promote staff members—include their pictures, pets, and community activities to help bond staff and clients to the practice.

Equine practices use a "winterize your horse" newsletter in the fall to reinforce the need for worming or teeth floating—two procedures most horse owners know and understand. Companion-animal practices use a newsletter to share the knowledge about spread of heartworms, giardia, or "traveling with your pet" concerns (over 50% of dog owners took their pet on vacation with them in 1999).

Make sure you have extra copies printed to use as handouts when you give talks. Give copies to new clients and others who come into your practice.

31. Do I need a logo?

A logo is a good idea. It's a symbol that announces: "This is us!" Make it simple so that it is easily recognizable by clients. The logo should be an expression of your practice's personality, and it should help you to stand out from the pack. Use it on everything: your sign, Yellow Pages ad, business cards, brochures, client handouts, invoices, prescription labels, name tags, and more. This is how you achieve full value from your logo.

32. Do I need a practice brochure?

Traditional practice brochures came into vogue in the 1980s. At that time they were little more than brag sheets and had a mixed reception. In the 1990s, we finally started to understand that the brochure is not a client rule book. Rather, it's a marketing tool for encouraging potential clients to come to the practice. Therefore, yes, you probably should have a practice brochure.

Develop it from a client's perspective. Many use a folder with looseleaf sheets rather than a brochure, so they can customize it and easily update inserts. The cover should show your hospital's name, logo, address, phone number, and emergency number. If you have a mission statement, the inside cover or first pocket is a good place to display it. Fill folders with information that pertains only to that owner and the pet(s) that was discussed in the consultation room. This makes each client feel special and increases the chances for a return visit.

You'll also have general pieces that talk about your veterinarians and staff, but even these should be inserts so that they can be easily changed and updated. Add a digitized photo of the pet to the insert pages to delight clients and increase personalization.

33. How can I make my reminder cards more effective?

The number one way to improve reminder cards is to send them on a regular basis. Make sure you are sending them for everything. For instance, do you send reminders for dental appointments and lab test appointments to monitor chronic diseases?

The more personalized the card, the better: "It's time for Bear's vaccinations," should become, "It's time for Bear's annual Life Cycle Consultation so that we can discuss his wellness needs for the coming year."

Always remember the **five-exposure rule**. When clients know they need to do it, it takes five exposures to get a "yes," so always give clients another chance. If you don't hear from them in 2 weeks, send a second reminder card. If you don't hear from the client after two mailings, call to find out if there is a problem. Do not ask why they did not come in. Rather, inquire in general terms, such as, "The doctor and I missed you and Bear this week. Is everything okay at your house?"

34. Is there really a senior's market?

It's no secret to marketers that active seniors are a lucrative market for many products and services. They have a fixed income, but their discretionary spending generally is far more flexible than that of a growing family with child demands.

There are more women (137.2 million) of all ages in the U.S. population than men (131.6 million), and the ratio of women to men increases dramatically with age. At ages 65 and over, there are 20.1 million women and 14.1 million men. At ages 85 and over, there are 2.8 million women vs. 1.1 million men. Among these women who are 65 and older, in 1997 almost half were widows and about 7 in 10 of these women lived alone.

The local senior citizen newspaper often is their primary communication means, except for those communities with a senior's center. Volunteer to write a regular pet care column or offer to come and speak to their monthly meeting. The bond will grow!

9. SUCCESSION PLANNING

SEPARATION OF ASSETS AND RESOURCES

1. What is succession planning?

In 1997, one of the authors (Catanzaro) started talking about "succession planning" in lieu of "buy-sell" requirements. Many have copied him in short order. The term succession planning describes the **evolution of practice ownership**, rather than just the transfer of funds and operational accountability. Succession planning is a process of social, legal, verbal, and inferred agreements that is required to develop expectations as well as keep promises with everyone involved with a business entity. In our case, a business entity is the entire veterinary practice, which includes staff, doctors, clients, bankers, families and friends.

Succession planning requires the nurturing and development of a practice team, so that continued employment is possible for everyone involved in the practice operations.

2. When do I start succession planning?

• When you have decided that your practice is mature, and you want to share the operational accountability with someone else.

• When you have exceeded the local lending limit and know that you will need to carry "paper" to sell the practice.

• When getting up and going to the practice does not make you feel special, professional, and wonderful.

• When you have reached 50 years of age and realize you have forgotten family, friends, and hobbies. The self-talk panic says, "There must be more to life than this!"

3. What is the actual succession planning process?

First, it may be a "buy-sell" thought. Then it becomes a transition of operational leadership, with shares of the practice being exchanged for accountability. The impetus for succession planning is a desire to step back from the daily grind and ensure that someone else is there to keep the practice moving forward.

Planning involves identifying a "partner" for the practice in the broadest terms. In today's market, the building and land are segregated into separate legal entities so that the new practice leader does not have to buy the dirt and building until after equity has been built.

4. What does "separation of assets and resources" mean?

Step one: Take the building and land out of the practice and establish a family LLC/LLP. You also may wish to establish an equipment trust, to allow payment of full-market-value lease cost to the entity (LLC/LLP) without a taxation concern for the practice.

Step two: Establish the legal entity for the practice, one that provides a liability shelter as well as a shareholder method that allows stair-step buy-in potential for future buyers.

Step three: Account for the feelings of the staff. Do not ask the staff to choose between the new and old. The practice transition must be smooth.

SLOWING DOWN YOUR LIFE—NOT YOUR PRACTICE

5. How do I slow down my life without damaging the practice?

- Know why you are "slowing down" your life. In recent years, many practices have been built on a balanced lifestyle desire.
- What will you do with the time if you have it? Is there something as important as the practice beckoning to you?
- Clients must be bonded *to the practice*—not a specific doctor—for a smooth transition when expanding or starting a succession plan. Therefore, increase the use of outpatient and inpatient nurses for client education and followup.
- When adding a doctor, always increase client access. Additional access may be outpatient hours during lunch, longer hours after supper, extended Saturday hours, or even more surgery, drop-off, or inpatient care time.

PASSING ON THE HEALTHCARE TEAM LEADERSHIP

6. How do I pass on the healthcare team leadership?

The best place to start is to share your leadership immediately. Quarterly, program-based budget reviews should involve all doctors and managers. Include a lead receptionist, coordinating receptionist, kennel master, lead outpatient nurse, and the inpatient nurse coordinator (i.e., those whom you trust on the staff).

Discussion of programs and procedures and evaluation of expected versus actual—not dollars—should be the "meat and potatoes" of the meeting. Commitment to programs is reflected in procedure counts and ratios (e.g., outpatient to dental, surgery and dental to anesthesia rates). Never assign blame; instead, make commitments to improve the future.

Many people have the titles but not the responsibility or authority to commit resources to achieve the end result. If you want to share leadership, clearly assign outcome expectations, discuss limitations and milestones, release the control of resources to the program manager, and stand back. Become a mentor, and do not try to control the process. Let the people try their way as long as it is within the original parameters and limitations. Be waiting at each milestone to ask, "Are we helping you enough to reach your objective? and "Can we provide additional assistance to help you achieve our goals in this race?"

RETIREMENT CONCERNS

7. What is the best way to address retirement concerns?

Start retirement planning the very first day you open the practice. Put 10% away every day, every week, and every month for retirement. Compounded money is very beneficial for retirement accounts.

Start diversification early. Separate the practice from the building and land by establishing two separate legal entities. Deal with each entity as a separate business. Expand real estate holdings concurrently with expanding the practice. Invest in real estate, mutual funds, and community bonds.

Never plan to sell the practice for retirement money. The sale of the practice should be your "mad money" at retirement. A good financial planner can assist your investment planning, just as a good practice consultant can assist your business growth.

10. AND THEN THERE IS TOMORROW . . .

FAMILIES AND FRIENDS ARE FOREVER

1. What is "balance" for a veterinary practice member?

Balance is developing a mix of the following elements, so that each day a smile greets you in the mirror, there is a spring in your step, and you are excited about participating in the world. If this energy has been lost, revisit these elements and regain those things that make life worth living for you.

An owner gets monetary pay from his or her practice in four areas: (1) clinical salary, (2) management fees, (3) return on investment, and (4) a share of excess net (money earned beyond the program-based budget forecast). An associate (and many owners) gets "paid" from (1) personal production, (2) pride in performance, (3) client gratitude, and (4) puppy breath.

The "inner self" grows by giving to others, whether it be rotary clubs, scouting, church, or other civic organizations. Developing relationships with a significant other and friends and/or pursuing family harmony expands the inner self even further.

The mind and body are recharged by sports, hobbies, theater, movies, reading, and related "unwind" activities.

2. Why families and friends? Why tomorrow?

Secret number 1: Unfortunately, tomorrow never comes, it just becomes today. Often tomorrow is too late, or at least that has been the case for the majority of veterinarians over the years. About half the marriages end in divorce, so strive to make yours the exception. Also spend time cultivating friendships.

Secret number 2: There must be something beyond veterinary practice, yet we see ketamine hydrochloride overdoses and substance abuse increasing, even at the student level. The perspective is out of focus for these people, and that is a sad story. Keep a clear idea of why you got into this profession in the first place—for the animals.

Secret number 3: "Get a life" means just that. Find a hobby, community service, family outing, personal activity, or something else that excites you as much as veterinary medicine. Always keep it in your weekly schedule!

IT'S ALL IN THE BALANCE

3. What offsets the lower wages in this field of medicine?
Staff and doctors alike believe veterinary medicine is their **personal calling**, which is why everyone works for such low wages. Technicians have a high drop-out rate, and new graduates are dropping out faster than the old curmudgeons because they want a balanced life, too. Raising a salary 50¢ per hour is about $1000 dollars a year; any practice can afford that. Start offering a livable wage!

4. How can I help practice members lead balanced lives?
A personal calling is noteworthy and significant for the individual who has found it, but not necessarily for those who support the individual. This is the balance—**caring for others**—that is needed. Never ask a parent to choose between family and veterinary medicine; you will immediately lose the loyalty of that person and may even drive him or her away.

The new generation of veterinary staff, doctors and paraprofessionals alike, consider their family and outside activity time as sacred elements of their lifestyle. Do not fight this; nurture it!

5. How can I determine if my life is balanced?
Of the people you sustain personal relationships with:
• Count those who will not talk veterinary medicine when you go out to dinner together (yes, you should be dining out weekly, looking for new client relations staff for your fast-growing practice).
• Count those with whom you have started to network for community improvements *not* related to animals.
• Count those who share your avocation, hobby, sport interest, and with whom you meet at least monthly to pursue those nonvocational interests.
• Count your staff members, including part-time. One face equals one count. If this count exceeds the above three, you need to get a grip on your lifestyle and balance your life immediately!
• Count the number of outings, dinners, etc. that you've scheduled during your personal time, and ask yourself, does this number allow balance in my life?

EFFICACY, EFFICIENCY, AND EFFECTIVENESS

6. What are the components of a better tomorrow?
1. An increase in clients; if 10% of total transactions are new clients, then the companion-animal practice is healthy.

2. Scheduling of two consultation rooms per doctor, with an outpatient nurse team, rather than scheduling of doctors in one column.

3. An appropriate fee schedule and client-access rate that allows about 43% of the gross to provide a good wage (W-2) to the staff and doctors.

4. Adequate facility space to hold and monitor animals so that the outpatient access and inpatient services are not reduced or limited due to congestion, smell, or other crowing factors.

5. A known set of *inviolate* core values that fits the practice team and the community. These have caused the succession plan to be accepted by those arriving as well as those phasing down, and have created team pride on a daily basis.

6. A balanced life, so that there is something "out there" besides veterinary medicine and the practice.

7. What are good efficiency measures for practice operations?

In healthcare, we strive for **efficacy**, not efficiency. Clients do not want an efficiency that makes them feel like a number, with no importance. The practice is effective if:

• clients have peace of mind while you are pursuing your diagnostics or treatment.

• the veterinary healthcare is **the right care for the right reason at the right price.** The price is a factor of client education and staff pride. The client must perceive that more was gained than just what was paid for during the process.

• the client returns to the practice at the desired time. It doesn't really matter if you cured the patient (efficiently or not) if the client never returns because a trust was violated.

Efficacy in life means achieving balance and knowing that when the time comes to write something on your tombstone, it will be a hard choice among the many contributions you have made to family, friends, and community.

APPENDIX A:

VETERINARY MANAGEMENT SOUND BITES FOR SUCCESS

All men are *not* created equal . . . over half are women!

No client is worse than *no* client.

Doctors deal in *needs*, not recommendations and soft hints.

When in doubt, the front door must swing!

While doctors produce gross, the staff earns the practice its net.

The only way to control chaos is to create it!

The secret is in the questions, not in the answers.

There are always more alternatives.

How you treat your staff is how your staff will treat your clients.

Give people more than they expect, and do it cheerfully.

Too many people overvalue what they are not and undervalue what they are.

When you say, "I'm sorry," look the person in the eye.

Directive training starts the delegation process; then persuasion and coaching are required to build the confidence needed to accept delegation.

Hire for attitude; train for skills and knowledge.

The greatest mistake is to imagine that we never will err.

Never laugh at anyone's dreams.

In disagreements, fight fairly. No name calling. Disagree, but do not make the other person wrong!

Don't judge people by their relatives.

Talk slowly, but think quickly.

When someone asks you a question you don't want to answer, smile and ask, "Why do you want to know?"

The art of using moderate abilities to advantage often brings greater results than actual brilliance.

Call you mother just to say "Hi, I love you."

When you lose, don't lose the lesson.

Remember the three Rs of staff development: respect for self and others; responsibility for all your actions; and recognition of the effort of others.

Don't let a little dispute injure a great friendship.

When you realize you've made a mistake, take immediate steps to correct it, and ask, "What can we do better next time?"

Smile when picking up the phone. The caller will hear it in your voice.

Spend some time alone.

Open your arms to change, but don't let go of your values.

Remember that silence is sometimes the best answer.

A *smart* veterinary business person is one who makes a mistake, learns from it, and never makes it again. A *wise* veterinary business person is one who finds a smart veterinary business person and learns from him or her how to avoid the mistakes.

Live a good, honorable life. Then when you get older and think back, you'll get to enjoy it a second time.

A caring atmosphere in your practice is so important. Do all you can to create a nurturing, harmonious practice environment.

In disagreements with others, deal with the current situation; don't bring up the past. Look to future behavior changes for all parties.

He who bravely dares must sometimes risk a fall.

Share your knowledge. It's a way to achieve immortality.

Nothing draws a crowd like a crowd.

Be careful of black-tongued dogs.

Time and money are interchangeable. You can always save one by spending more of the other.

Mind your own business.

Once a year, go someplace you've never been before.

Put 10% of every earned dollar immediately into investments. If you make a lot of money, put it to use helping others while you are living; that is wealth's greatest satisfaction.

Remember that not getting what you want is sometimes a stroke of luck.

Learn the rules, then break some. Call it a test!

The client is an asset to protect.

Judge your success by what you had to give up to get it.

Continuous quality improvement is a habit that causes everyone to contribute to the practice success.

Approach love and cooking with reckless abandon.

Send someone to continuing education and require that one great idea gets unilaterally implemented by them for every day away from the practice.

Believe in others at first sight, share the practice core values, and nurture their efforts.

Remember that your character is your destiny.

Look with new eyes, and the ordinary and familiar become fresh.

Always examine the opposite point of view, even if you don't have opposition. You'll make better decisions.

Words are powerful. Call a problem an opportunity and you'll treat it like one.

Find five things to be grateful for everyday, and you life will get better.

Pet a puppy or kitten today. It's one of the perks of the job.

Don't sweat the small stuff . . . and it's all small stuff!

Read between the lines.

Health is more than just the absence of disease; it's a happy, vibrant life, doing the most with what you have, with delight.

Imagination is more important than knowledge.

Feel gratitude for living and show it through your actions. Help others who suffer.

Use it or lose it! Do not accumulate old equipment for your legacy museum; donate it and take the tax write-off.

Only a life lived for others is worthwhile.

Experience is not what happens to you, but what you *do* with what happens to you. If wisdom is a diamond, experience is a diamond mine.

Hope is a thing with feathers that perches in the soul.

There is a fine line between bravery and stupidity. If you get away with it, you are brave. If you don't, you are stupid.

The most fatal illusion is the settled point of view. Life is growth and motion.

A veterinarian's purpose is to give the client peace of mind while the disease takes its course in the patient.

Everyone has creative potential; the unique expression of yourself is the beginning.

Be part of the healing team; be positive about opportunities and challenges.

"What if I spent money on training an employee, and then they leave?" What if you don't, and they stay?

The person who says it cannot be done should not interrupt the person doing it.

There's never time to do it right, but there's always time to do it over.

Read more books, and watch less TV.

You're more likely to receive forgiveness than permission.

Try a thing you haven't done three times: once, to get over the fear of doing it; twice, to learn how to do it; and a third time to figure out whether you like it or not.

Profit is not a four-letter word.

Success = attitude + training + vision + procedure

A failure to plan is a plan to fail.

Plan your work. Work your plan.

None of us is as important as all of us.

You can't manage what you don't measure.

You can't expect what you don't inspect.

Management by intimidation brings compliance, but it does not bring commitment.

Don't believe all you hear, spend all you have, or sleep all you want.

Remember that great love and great achievements involve great risk.

Be gentle with the earth.

Have a life outside practice. Love deeply and passionately. You might get hurt, but it's the only way to live life completely.

You can teach someone to talk nice, but you can't teach someone to *be* nice!

Never interrupt when you are being flattered.

The only real mistake you can make is not to learn from your mistakes.

To the world you might be one person, but to one person you might be the world.

Real friends are those who, when you feel you've made a fool of yourself, don't think you've done a permanent job.

Sometimes the majority only means that all the fools are on the same side.

I don't have to attend every argument I'm invited to.

Lead your life so you won't be ashamed to sell the family parrot to the town gossip.

People gather bundles of sticks to build bridges they never cross.

Life is 10% of what happens to you, and 90% of how you respond to it.

Life is like an onion; you peel off one layer at a time, and sometimes you weep.

Learn from the mistakes of others. You can't live long enough to make them all yourself.

Following the path of least resistance is what makes rivers and men crooked.

When it comes time to die . . . make sure all you have left to do is die.

APPENDIX B:

GLOSSARY OF TERMS

(or "A Rose By Any Other Name . . . Is Confusing!")

A

AAHA: American Animal Hospital Association

AAVMC: American Association of Veterinary Medical Colleges

absolute rigid flexibility: a mindset that allows changes and fine tuning during implementation to make a plan work better

accountability: an organizational obligation held by a team member, generally with a clearly defined outcome.

ACHE: American College of Healthcare Executives

ACT: average client transaction

active listening: the conscious effort to secure information of all kinds; involves giving the speaker full attention, listening intently and being alert to any clues of spoken or unspoken meaning or resistance, and actively seeking to keep the conversation open and satisfying to the speaker

adminis-trivia: catch-phrase for administrative trivia

appraisal interview: a meeting held between a supervisor and an employee to review the performance rating and, using that evaluation as a basis, to discuss the overall quality of the employee's work and methods for improving it, if necessary; should be replaced by performance planning once CQI is understood

authority: the legitimate power to direct people to work for the good of the practice; can make resources available so that employees can achieve desired outcomes

AVMA: American Veterinary Medical Association

B

behavior: the actions people take, or the things they say, while coping with other people, problems, opportunities, and situations

benchmarking: otherwise known as brain-picking; using all the brains you can beg, borrow, or steal

body language: nonverbal body movements, facial expressions, or gestures that may project and reveal underlying attitudes and sentiments; may convey a message similar to, or different from, the words used

brainstorming: a group approach to idea generation that encourages free association of ideas among participants, forbids negative judgments, and creates a maximum number of ideas in a short period of time

budget: a planning and reporting system that incorporates many standards for operating programs and results, as well as for costs and expenses, into a single dynamic document

C

catchment area: primary geographical areas served by an institution; demographic area from which clients come

commitment: the individual team member's belief and investment in the practice's core values, his or her job role, and the feedback process

communication method: the form or technique by which information is communicated; includes attitude, performance, appearance, speech, demonstration, and deed

communication process: the verbal and nonverbal giving and receiving of information and understanding as a result of thinking, doing, observing, talking, listening, writing, and reading; exchange between two or more people, leading to a desired action or attitude

core values: personal standards of excellence and philosophy of operations that underlie all decisions; inviolate beliefs of a leader on which others also can depend

CQI: continuous quality improvement; embraces change in a never-ending quest for improved healthcare delivery

D

decision making: evaluating alternative solutions and making a choice among them; part of the problem-solving process

delegation: the assignment to others of organizational responsibilities or obligations along with appropriate practice authority, power, and rights

division of work: the principle that performance is more efficient when a large job is broken down into smaller, specialized jobs

E

employee-centered supervision: management emphasis on a genuine concern and respect for staff members as human beings and on maintaining effective relationships within a work group

employee counseling: a task oriented, problem solving technique that features an empathic, interactive discussion; emphasizes listening and is aimed at helping a team member cope with some specific aspect of his or her practice life

employee turnover: a measure of how many people come to work for an organization and do not remain employed by that organization, for whatever reason

F

facilitating: assisting and guiding others in their efforts to perform their jobs, rather than emphasizing orders and instructions

feedback: some return of the output of a mechanism, process, or system, as input; informative reaction or response

free association of ideas: the ability of the mind to unconsciously visualize relationships between seemingly different objects and ideas ("brain storming")

G

grapevine: informal network that staff members use to convey information of interest to them; fast, but lacks a high degree of accuracy and reliability

group dynamics: the interaction among members of a work group and concurrent changes in their attitudes, behavior, and relationships; similarly, the interaction between a work group and others outside the group

H

halo effect: a generalization whereby one aspect of performance, or a single quality of an individual's nature, is allowed to overshadow everything else about that person

healthcare: the medical, dental, or veterinary delivery of services, products, and empathy

HEAP: history, evaluation, assessment, plan; one way to organize medical records

human-relations management: an approach that seeks to stimulate cooperation via understanding of, and genuine concern for, staff members as individuals and as critical elements of a work group

I

infinity model: a leadership and management single-flow diagram; a process, not a program; starts as a total commitment by the leaders, and grows toward endless possibilities

inner strength: internal values and beliefs a person possesses that allow confidence and determination in outward activities

J

jargon: the technical terminology or characteristic idiom of a special activity or group; used within a practice team, but seldom appropriate for use with clients or outside the practice

job aids: materials on or near the work area to help employees remember key points (what to do and how to do it) and perform effectively

job role: the team member's part in the practice's operational environment

L

leader: someone who gives credit and takes blame; gets things done through other people

litigious: inclined toward involvement in lawsuits

M

management development: a systematic program to improve the knowledge, attitudes, and skills of supervisors and managers

manager: an individual who plans, organizes, directs, and controls the work of others in an organization

mentor: a knowledgeable, often influential, individual who takes an interest in, and advises, another person to assist in making them successful

mind mapping: obtaining as many "wild and crazy" ideas as possible in a short period of time

modeling: the process in which a skilled coworker or supervisor demonstrates the performance of a key job skill and simultaneously explains the steps involved and the reasons for doing them; in management, also a graphic representation of a system

motivation: highly individual needs for survival, security, companionship, respect, achievement, power, growth, and personal worth that impel a person to behave in a certain manner

O

objectives: also referred to as goals and standards; the short-term and long-term targets toward which an organization strives

ogre: the doctor after a 22-hour shift

outer strength: elements of management and personality that are displayed to others in the practice's operational environment

P

participation: the technique by which team members share work-related information, responsibilities, and/or decisions; may be used to determine the way a job should be performed, how a group should divide up the work, and what work goals should be

patient advocate: one who speaks for the animal's needs, rather than uses fear tactics to push a "sale"

performance appraisal: a formal and outdated evaluation system to grade how well a person is performing and measure his or her work to a static standard; in healthcare, replaced by CQI and performance planning

performance planning: a dynamic process in which 90-day goals and the measure(s) of success are jointly agreed upon by an individual and his or her mentor, then implemented; includes evaluation of efforts both during and after the 90-day training period.

personality: an individual's unique way of behaving and interpreting the actions of other people and events; shaped by heredity, parents' beliefs, upbringing, work experiences, and many other factors

policies: broad guidelines, philosophy, or principles established by a practice to support its organizational goals

practice owner: in charge of and responsible for the performance of the team; establishes broad plans, objectives, and general policies

proactive: using previous learning, recall, and tenacity to prevent or resolve a challenge *before* others can become reactionary

problem solving: when expectations don't match actual conditions or results, the process whereby the situation is analyzed systematically to find and remedy its causes

procedures: minimum standards prescribed by management for proper and consistent sequences and channels of work flow *productivity:* the measure of effectiveness that compares the value of outputs from an operation with the cost of the resources used

program-based budget: expense compared with income for same line items, or specific program income compared with outpatient visits, or any other number of dynamic ratios. This varies from practice to practice.

purpose: most often defined in terms of values, mission, and/or philosophy within the practice; the hub around which all else evolves to make the team effective and focused

Q

quality assurance: establishing milestones and outcome accountabilities for a plan and spot-checking measurements of success toward the end result(s)

quality control: an aggregate of activities designed to ensure that a process is followed with a high degree of consistency

quality of work life: the idea that work must be psychologically and spiritually, as well as materially, rewarding

quick fix: an expedient, often inadequate, solution to a problem

R

regulations: special rules, orders, and controls set by an authority to restrict the conduct of individuals or organizations

responsibility: a duty or obligation to perform a prescribed task or service or to attain a specified objective

S

satisfaction: the state that exists when truly motivating factors are provided, such as interesting and challenging work, full use of one's capabilities, and recognition for achievement

SOAP: subjective, objective, assessment, plan; one way of organizing medical records

stasis: act or condition of standing or stopping; in healthcare, it equals stagnation

stress: on- or off-job pressures that place a burden on an individual's physical, mental, and nervous system

succession planning: the evolution of practice ownership

supervisor: manager or coordinator in charge of the activities of a group; directs work procedures, issues oral and written orders and instructions, assigns duties to workers, examines work for quality and neatness, maintains harmony among workers, and adjusts errors and complaints

synergy: combined action or force that is greater than one element

system: an interrelated set of elements that function as a whole

T

TQM: total quality management; improvement movement in industry

TQS/TMS: total quality service/total management service; "copy-cat" management ideas of lateral organizations trying to reinvent TQM/CQI

U

unity of direction: the principle that there should be a set of goals and objectives that unifies the activities of everyone in an organization

V

values: a set of personal beliefs that form the foundation for life decisions

W

work: that four-letter word for employment; provides the means to pay the bills

Some terms were adapted from Bittel LR, Newstrom JW: What Every Supervisor Should Know, 6th ed. New York, McGraw-Hill, 1990.

APPENDIX C:

STAFF TRAINING & ORIENTATION FORMS

SAMPLE NEW RECEPTIONIST ORIENTATION CHECKLIST

Phase I—Organizational (1 week)   Expected completion date _____

During your first week on the team, you will learn the basic structure of this team and identify the individual personal strengths. During this phase you will be expected to:

1. Meet all other staff members _____

2. Complete the required forms:
   personnel information _____
   form I-9 _____
   form W-4 _____
   radiation badge request (if applicable) _____

3. Become familiar with the location of all hospital work areas _____

4. Learn how to complete time cards and the location of the time clock _____

5. Learn where bulletin boards and work schedules are posted _____

6. Review the Hospital Safety Manual to be able to:
   activate the fire alarm _____
   locate the fire extinguishers and emergency exits
      in your work area _____
   locate the MSDS for common chemicals
      in your work area _____
   locate the emergency eye wash station(s)
      in your work area _____
   review the safety workbook and complete
      the self-assessment test _____

7. Become familiar with the location of supplies _____

8. Become familiar with the uniform/dress code _____

9. Become familiar with the organizational structure of the hospital _____

10. Learn the hospital schedule for meals and breaks _____

11. Learn payday procedures and overtime policy _____

12. Receive your personal copy of the Staff Policy Manual _____

13. Adhere to client information and confidentiality rules _____

14. Read the Hospital Housekeeping Manual and be able to perform the tasks assigned to your position _____

15. Learn the hospital medical record filing system _____

16. Provide feedback to your supervisor about the process of orientation and the ideas and techniques learned during this phase of your training _____

17. Complete the computer tutorial training program _____

18. View the following AAHA training films and workbooks:
    Telephone Techniques _____
    First Impressions _____
    Special Situations _____

Phase II—Introduction (2 weeks)   Expected completion date _____

During your 2nd and 3rd weeks on the team, you must use effective communication techniques to define the characteristics and needs of the new team. During this phase you will be expected to:

1. Learn to answer the telephone cheerfully and promptly _____

2. Learn to give directions to the hospital _____

3. Learn to properly and completely relay messages _____

4. Learn the hospital's appointment and patient handling systems _____

5. Learn the necessary record keeping requirements for:
    routine outpatient check-in procedures _____
    routine outpatient check-out procedures _____
    inpatient check-in procedures _____
    inpatient check-out procedures _____
    day care/drop-off check-in procedures _____
    day care/drop-off check-out procedures _____
    boarding check-in procedures _____
    boarding check-out procedures _____

6. Learn the hospital's common client handouts _____

7. Learn basic medical terminology _____

8. Learn the hospital's heartworm information and preventatives _____

Appendix C 151

9. Learn to update client records at each contact for:
    current name, address, phone, work phone, etc. _____
    patient name, weight, vaccination status _____
    status of heartworm prevention & test _____
    surgical neutering if applicable _____
    recording client complaint/request _____

10. Learn the hospital's vaccination protocols _____

11. Learn the hospital's basic fee schedule and how
    to look up nonroutine procedures or products _____

12. Learn how to input recalls, rechecks, and reminders _____

13. Learn the city and county licensing requirements _____

14. Learn to issue/reissue rabies/license tags/certificates _____

15. Learn proper techniques for collecting:
    cash _____
    checks _____
    credit card payments _____

16. Provide feedback to your supervisor about the process
    of orientation and the ideas and techniques learned
    during this phase of your training _____

17. Learn to process returned merchandise _____

18. View the following training films:
    How to care for your new puppy _____
    Canine parvovirus enteritis _____
    Cats and their health _____
    Canine vaccinations _____
    Feline vaccinations _____
    Canine heartworm disease _____

Phase III—Basic Skills (3 weeks)   **Expected completion date** _____

During your 4th through 6th weeks on the team, you will begin to reflect on the new dynamics of the team and to represent the needs of the group in everyday activities. During this phase you will be expected to:

1. Learn the end-of-day closing procedures _____

2. Learn the start-of-day opening procedures _____

3. Begin performing client recalls for missed appointments _____

152   Appendix C

4. Learn to process client refunds   _____
5. Learn to process nonsufficient funds (NSF) checks from bank   _____
6. Learn the location of other local animal service businesses   _____
7. Learn to prepare bank deposits   _____
8. Learn to receive and direct incoming mail/packages   _____
9. Learn to process requests for prescription refills   _____
10. Learn to receive results from the reference lab   _____
11. Learn to educate the client about common surgical procedures,
    e.g., no food or water the morning of surgery, basic description
    of procedure   _____
12. Learn to process medical emergencies   _____
13. Provide feedback to your supervisor about the process
    of orientation and the ideas and techniques learned during
    this phase of your training   _____
14. View the following training films:
    AAHA Advanced Veterinary Receptionist   _____

Phase IV—Advanced Skills (6 weeks)   Expected completion date _____

During your 7th through 12th weeks on the team, you will begin to perform solo tasks based on your knowledge of the team's resources. You now have a better understanding of the "big picture" of the operation. During this phase you will be expected to:

1. Reflect on previous tasks that you have still not mastered
   and re-cycle them into this phase   _____
2. Learn to complete reminders, sympathy cards, etc.   _____
3. Learn NSF check redemption procedures   _____
4. Learn computer back-up procedures   _____
5. Learn to complete paperwork for petty cash reimbursement   _____
6. Learn to inactivate client/patient files   _____
7. Learn to conduct accounts receivable followups   _____
8. Learn the computer maintenance procedures:
   daily   _____
   weekly   _____

monthly _____
yearly _____

9. Provide feedback to your supervisor about the process of orientation and the ideas and techniques learned during this phase of your training _____

10. View the following AAHA training films and workbooks:
    Understanding Client Pet Loss _____
    Counseling Clients _____
    The Loss of Your Pet _____

SAMPLE NEW TECHNICIAN/ASSISTANT ORIENTATION CHECKLIST

Phase I—Organizational (1 week)   **Expected completion date** _____

During your first week on the team, you will learn the basic structure of this team and identify the individual personal strengths. During this phase you will be expected to:

1. Meet all other staff members _____

2. Complete the required forms:
   personnel information
   form I-9 _____
   form W-4 _____
   radiation badge request _____

3. Become familiar with the location of all hospital work areas _____

4. Learn how to complete time cards and the location of the time clock _____

5. Learn where bulletin boards and work schedules are posted _____

6. Review the Hospital Safety Manual and be able to:
   activate the fire alarm _____
   locate the fire extinguishers and emergency exits
     in your work area _____
   locate the MSDS for common chemicals
     in your work area _____
   locate the emergency eye wash station(s)
     in your work area _____
   review the safety workbook and complete the
     self-assessment test _____

154   Appendix C

7. Become familiar with the location of supplies   _____

8. Become familiar with the uniform/dress code   _____

9. Become familiar with the organizational structure
   of the hospital   _____

10. Learn the hospital schedule for meals and breaks   _____

11. Learn payday procedures and overtime policy   _____

12. Receive your personal copy of the Staff Policy Manual   _____

13. Adhere to client information and confidentiality rules   _____

14. Read the Hospital Housekeeping Manual and be able
    to perform the tasks assigned to your position   _____

15. Provide feedback to your supervisor about the process
    of orientation and the ideas and techniques learned
    during this phase of your training   _____

16. View the following training films:
    How to care for your new puppy   _____
    Canine parvovirus enteritis   _____
    Cats and their health   _____
    Canine vaccinations   _____
    Feline vaccinations   _____
    Canine heartworm disease   _____

Phase II—Introduction (2 weeks)   Expected completion date _____

During your 2nd and 3rd weeks on the team, you must use effective communication techniques to define the characteristics and needs of the new team. During this phase you will be expected to:

1. Properly answer the telephone or greet clients when the receptionist
   is unable to   _____

2. Learn the hospital's medical record filing system   _____

3. Learn the hospital's common medical abbreviations   _____

4. Learn basic medical terminology   _____

5. Properly clean and disinfect cages and runs   _____

6. Prepare meals for hospitalized patients and boarders   _____

7. Properly sanitize food and water pans   _____

Appendix C   155

8. Learn the medical waste disposal procedures   _____
9. Begin recording data on patients' appetites, excretions, etc.   _____
10. Begin performing baths and dips   _____
11. Learn how to obtain stool samples   _____
12. Learn how to obtain/record patients' vital signs   _____
13. Learn how to prepare samples for inhouse lab testing   _____
14. Learn how to prepare samples for reference lab testing   _____
15. Restrain animals correctly for all procedures   _____
16. Learn how to remove a frightened animal from a cage/run   _____
17. Learn how to apply a hasty muzzle   _____
18. Learn the proper use and care of clippers, blades, etc.   _____
19. Learn how to prepare and label medications for dispensing   _____
20. Learn the necessary record-keeping requirements for:
    dispensing/administering controlled substances   _____
    admitting patients for hospitalization/boarding/daycare   _____
    performing veterinarian-directed treatments   _____
21. Provide feedback to your supervisor about the process of orientation and the ideas and techniques learned during this phase of your training   _____
22. View the following AAHA video training tapes and workbooks:
    Medication Administration   _____
    Animal Restraint & Handling   _____

Phase III—Basic Nursing Skills (3 weeks)
Expected completion date _____

During your 4th through 6th weeks on the team, you will begin to reflect on the new dynamics of the team and to represent the needs of the group in everyday activities. During this phase you will be expected to:

1. Properly trim patients' nails   _____
2. Properly clean patients' ears   _____
3. Properly express patients' anal glands   _____
4. Learn to identify and locate commonly used medications   _____
5. Properly prepare and read fecal and heartworm tests   _____

6. Prepare the correct vaccines for patients _____
7. Prepare fluids, IV dripset, and catheter for use _____
8. Properly flush IV catheters and change IV bags _____
9. Learn to properly add medication to IV drips _____
10. Properly prepare medications for IV, SQ, and IM administration _____
11. Learn to properly prepare patients for surgery _____
12. Learn to properly prepare the operatory for use _____
13. Learn to properly prepare and sterilize surgical packs:
    instrument packs _____
    gown packs _____
    towel/drape packs _____
    specialty packs _____
    cold sterilization trays _____
14. Learn to identify and care for common instruments _____
15. Learn how to properly prepare dental equipment for use _____
16. Learn how to properly perform dental prophylaxis _____
17. Learn how to safely and correctly prepare equipment for radiological procedures:
    use of monitoring badge _____
    use of personal protection equipment _____
    turning on machine _____
    placement of cassette _____
    use of collimator _____
    labeling/marking procedures _____
    use of calipers/measurement of target area _____
    use of technique chart _____
    setting of machine parameters _____
    completion of the exposure log _____
18. Provide feedback to your supervisor about the process of orientation and the ideas and techniques learned during this phase of your training _____
19. View the following AAHA video training tapes and workbooks:
    Fluid Administration _____
    Basic Radiology _____

Phase IV—Advanced Nursing (6 weeks)
Expected completion date _____

During your 7th through 12th weeks on the team, you will begin to perform solo tasks based on your knowledge of the team's resources. You now have a better understanding of the "big picture" of the operation. During this phase, you will be expected to:

1. Reflect on previous tasks that you have still not mastered and re-cycle them into this phase _____
2. Learn the location and use of emergency drugs _____
3. Learn the proper administration of emergency drugs _____
4. Begin performing dental prophylaxis _____
5. Learn to properly administer IM, SQ, and IV injections _____
6. Learn how to properly collect hematology samples for:
   heartworm filter/antigen tests _____
   CBC w/differential _____
   serum chemistry panel _____
7. Learn how to properly perform ECG _____
8. Learn the hospital's recommendations for clients regarding:
   estrous and breeding cycles of dogs and cats _____
   proper nutrition for dogs and cats _____
   parasite screening and prevention _____
   heartworm disease transmission, testing, and prevention _____
   flea control on pets and in the house and yard _____
   surgical neutering of dogs and cats _____
   vaccination protocol for dogs and cats _____
9. Learn the techniques for intubation of patients _____
10. Learn how to identify the stages and planes of anesthesia _____
11. Begin monitoring of anesthetized patients _____
12. Begin performing radiographic procedures independently _____
13. Begin performing inhouse laboratory procedures independently _____
14. Provide feedback to your supervisor about the process of orientation and the ideas and techniques learned during this phase of your training _____

15. View the following AAHA video training tapes and workbooks:
    Dental Prophylaxis   _____
    Bereavement Counseling   _____

APPENDIX D:

READING LIST

VETERINARY SPECIFIC READING

Boss, Nan. *Educating Your Clients from A . . . to Z: What to Say and How to Say It.* AAHA, Denver, Colorado, 1999.

Catanzaro, Thomas E. *Building the Successful Veterinary Practice: Leadership Tools.* Vol. 1. Ames, Iowa, ISUP, 1997.

Catanzaro, Thomas E. *Building the Successful Veterinary Practice: Programs and Procedures.* Vol. 2. Ames, Iowa, Iowa State University Press (ISUP), 1997.

Catanzaro, Thomas E. *Building the Successful Veterinary Practice: Innovation and Creativity.* Vol. 3. Ames, Iowa, ISUP, 1998.

Catanzaro, Thomas E. *Design Starter Kit for Veterinary Hospitals*, 3rd ed. Denver, Colorado, AAHA, 1996.

Catanzaro, Thomas E. *Veterinary Management in Transition: Preparing for the 21st Century.* Ames, Iowa, ISUP, 2000.

Catanzaro, Thomas E., et al. *Beyond the Successful Veterinary Practice: Succession Planning and Other Legal Issues.* Ames, Iowa, ISUP, 2000.

Catanzaro, Thomas E., et al. *Veterinary Healthcare Services: Options in Delivery.* Ames, Iowa, ISUP, 2000.

Fassig, Samuel M., et al. *Veterinary Associates Survival Guide.* Denver, Colorado, AAHA, 2000.

Finch, Lloyd. *Telephone Courtesy & Client Service.* Menlo Park, California, AVMA, Crisp Publications, 1987.

Gerson, Richard F. *Beyond Customer Service: Keeping Clients for Life.* Menlo Park, California, AVMA, Crisp Publications, 1994.

Haberer, JoAnn B., and Marylou Wendel Webb. *Teamwork: 50 Ways to Make it Work in Your Practice.* Menlo Park, California, AVMA, Crisp Publications, 1996.

Jevring, Caroline. *Managing a Veterinary Practice.* London, W.B. Saunders, 1996.

Jevring, Caroline, and Thomas Catanzaro. *Healthcare of the Well Pet.* W.B. Saunders, 1999.

Lagoni, Laurel, and Dana Durrance. *Connecting with Clients: Practical Communication Techniques for 15 Common Situations.* Denver, Colorado, AAHA, undated.

Scott, Dru. *Client Satisfaction: The Other Half of Your Job.* Los Altos, California, AVMA, Crisp Publications, 1988.

BEST BUSINESS READING

Bennis, Warren, and Bert Nanus. *Leaders, Strategies for Taking Charge.* New York, Harper and Row, 1985.

Block, Peter. *The Empowered Manager: Positive Political Skills at Work.* San Francisco, Jossey-Bass, 1987.

Case, John. *Open-Book Management: The Coming Business Revolution.* New York, Harper Collins, 1996.

Peters, Tom. *Liberation Management: Necessary Disorganization for the Nanosecond Nineties.* New York, Knopf, 1992.

Senge, Peter M. *The Fifth Discipline: The Art and Practice of the Learning Organization.* New York, Doubleday, 1990.

Successful Financial Management. Denver, Colorado, AAHA, 1987.

COMMUNICATION

Bazerman, Max H., and Margaret A. Neale. *Negotiating Reality.* New York, Free Press, 1992.

Decker, Bert, with Jim Denney. *You've Got to Be Believed to Be Heard.* New York, St. Martin's, 1992.

Frank, Milo O. *How to Get Your Point Across in Thirty Seconds.* New York, Simon and Schuster, 1986.

McCallister, Linda. *I Wish I'd Said That: How to Talk Your Way Out of Trouble and into Success.* New York, Wiley, 1992.

Mosvick, K., and Robert B. Nelson. *We've Got to Start Meeting Like This: A Guide to Successful Business Meeting Management.* Glenview, IL, Scott Foresman, 1987.

Rafe, Stephen C. *How to Be Prepared to Think on Your Feet.* New York, Harper Business, 1990.

GET READY FOR TOMORROW

Drucker, Peter F. *Managing for the Future: The 1990s and Beyond.* New York, Dutton, 1992.

Drucker, Peter F. *Post Capitalistic Society.* New York, Harper Collins, 1993.

Dychtwald, Ken, and Joe Flower. *Age Wave: The Challenges and Opportunities of an Aging America.* Los Angeles, J. P. Tarcher, 1989.

Jamieson, David, and Julie O'Mara. *Managing Workforce 2000: Gaining the Diversity Advantage.* San Francisco, Jossey-Boss, 1991.

McNally, David. *Even Eagles Need a Push.* New York, Bantam Doubleday Dell, 1990.

Schwartz, Peter. *The Art of the Long View.* New York, Doubleday, 1991.

LEADERSHIP SKILLS

Atchison, T.A. *Turning Healthcare Leadership Around.* San Francisco, Jossey-Bass, 1991.

Boone, Mary E. *Leadership and the Computer.* Rocklin, CA, Prima, 1991.

Carnegie, Dale. *The Leader in You.* New York, Simon and Schuster, 1993.

Covey, Stephen R. *Seven Habits of Highly Effective People.* New York, Simon and Schuster, Fireside, 1990.

Drucker, Peter F. *Managing for Results: Economic Tasks and Risk-Taking.* New York, Harper and Row, 1964.

Juran, J.M. *Juran on Leadership for Quality.* New York, Free Press, 1989.

Pagonis, William G. *Moving Mountains.* Waco, TX, Baylor Univ Extract, 1985.

LEARNING TO MOTIVATE PEOPLE

Albrecht, Karl, with Steven Albrecht. *The Creative Corporation.* Homewood, IL, Dow Jones-Irwin, 1987.

Costello, Bill. *Awaken Your Birdbrain.* Bowie, MD, Thinkorporated, 1998.

Kravetz, Dennis J. *The Human Resources Revolution: Implementing Progressive Management Practices for Bottom-Line Success.* San Francisco, Jossey-Bass, 1988.

Levering, Robert. *A Great Place to Work.* New York, Random House, 1988.

Matejka, Ken E. *Why This Horse Won't Drink: How to Win and Keep Employee Commitment.* New York, American Management Association, 1991.

Roethlisberger, Fritz Jules. *Management and Morale.* Cambridge, MA, Harvard University Press, 1941.

von Oech, Roger. *A Kick in the Seat of the Pants.* New York, Harper and Row, Perennial Library, 1986.

MANAGEMENT SKILLS THAT WORK

Douglass, Merrill, et al. *Manage Your Time, Your Work, Yourself.* New York, AMACOM, 1993.

Jellison, Jerald M. *Overcoming Resistance: A Practical Guide to Producing Change in the Work Place.* New York, Simon and Schuster, 1993.

Kaplan, Robert E. *Beyond Ambition: How Driven Managers Can Lead Better and Live Better.* San Francisco, Jossey-Bass, 1991.

Katzenbach, Jon R., and Douglas K. Smith. *The Wisdom of Teams: Creating the High-Performance Organization.* Boston, Harvard Business School Press, 1993.

LeBoeuf, Michael. *The Greatest Management Principle in the World.* New York, Berkley Books, 1985.

NEW TACTICS FOR MANAGERS

Bardwick, Judith M. *Danger in the Comfort Zone: From Boardroom to Mailroom—How to Break the Entitlement Habit That's Killing American Business.* New York, AMACOM, 1991.

Bittel, Lester R., and John W. Newstrom. *What Every Supervisor Should Know,* 6th ed. New York, McGraw-Hill, 1990.

Horton, R., and Peter C. Reid. *Beyond the Trust Gap: Forging a New Partnership Between Managers and Their Employees.* Homewood, IL, Business One Irwin, 1991.

Leebov, Wendy, and Gail Scott. *Healthcare Managers in Transition.* San Francisco, Jossey-Bass, 1990.

Shonk, James H. *Team-Based Organization: Developing a Successful Team Environment.* Homewood, IL, Business One Irwin, 1992.

REACH YOUR CUSTOMERS

Albrecht, Karl, and Lawrence J. Bradford. *The Service Advantage: How to Identify and Fulfill Customer Needs.* Homewood, IL, Dow Jones-Irwin, 1990.

Carlzon, Jan. *Moments of Truth.* Cambridge, MA, Ballinger, 1987.

Connellan, Thomas K., and Ron Zemke. *Sustaining Knock-Your-Socks-Off Service.* New York, AMACOM, 1993.

Davidow, William H., and Bro Uttal. *Total Customer Service: The Ultimate Weapon.* New York, Harper and Row, 1989.

LeBoeuf, Michael. *How to Win Customers and Keep Them for Life.* New York, Berkley Books, 1987.

SHARPEN YOUR PERSONAL SKILLS

Bracey, Hyler, et al. *Managing from the Heart.* New York, Delacorte, 1990.

Gottlieb, Marvin, and William J. Healy. *Making Deals: The Business of Negotiating.* New York, New York Institute of Finance, 1990.

Heirs, Ben, with Peter Farrell. *The Professional Decision Thinker: America's New Management and Education Priority.* New York, Dodd Mead, 1987.

Nelson, Robert B. *Empowering Employees Through Delegation.* Burr-Ridge, IL, Irwin Professional Publications, 1994.

Seiwert, Lothar J. *Time Is Money: Save It.* Homewood, IL, Dow Jones-Irwin, 1989.

Webber, Ross Arkell. *Becoming a Courageous Manager: Overcoming Career Problems of New Managers.* Englewood Cliffs, NJ, Prentice Hall, 1991.

WINNING SALES TECHNIQUES

Hanan, Mack, *Successful Market Penetration: How to Shorten the Sales Cycle by Making the First Sale the First Time.* New York, American Management Association, 1987.

Laughlin, Chuck, et al. *Samurai Selling: The Ancient Art of Service in Sales.* New York, St. Martin's, 1993.

Willingham, Ron. *Integrity Selling: How to Succeed in Selling in the Competitive Years Ahead.* Garden City, NY, Doubleday, 1987.

Wilson, Larry, with Hersch Wilson. *Changing the Game: The New Way to Sell.* New York, Simon and Schuster, Fireside, 1988.

INDEX

Page numbers in **boldface type** indicate complete chapters.

AAHA. *See* American Animal Hospital Association
AAVMC. *See* American Association of Veterinary Medical Colleges
Absolute rigid flexibility, 141
Accidents, work-related, 79–81
Accountability
  definition of, 141
  operational, 127
Accountants, 17–18
Accounting, tax, 26
Accounting software, 26
ACE (Americans Communicating Electronically), 9
ACT (average client transaction), 14, 141
Active listening, 141
"Adminis-trivia," 141
Admonishment, letters of, 78
Advertising
  on the Internet
    for new associates, 105
    web pages, 28–29
  of new practices, 9, 10, 36
  "sell the sizzle" approach in, 46–47
  for staff recruitment, 44
  in the Yellow Pages, 36, 121
Alter ego doctrine, 109–111
Alternative medicine, 4
American Animal Hospital Association (AAHA)
  certification process of, public's lack of awareness of, 36
  Chart of Accounts of, 17, 26
  as "The Current and Future Market for Veterinarians and the Veterinary Medical Services in the United States" study sponsor, 1
  Design Start Kit for Veterinary Hospitals of, 12
  member hospitals, client referrals by, 36
  staff development multi-media tools of, 54
  Standards for Veterinary Hospitals of, 92
American Association of Veterinary Medical Colleges (AAVMC), as "The Current and Future Market for Veterinarians and the Veterinary Medical Services in the United States" study sponsor, 1
American Boarding Kennel Association, 99
American College of Healthcare Executives, 40, 141
Americans Communicating Electronically (ACE), 9
American Veterinary Medical Association (AVMA)
  American Veterinary Medical Foundation of, ClientLink video training program of, 54
  as "The Current and Future Market for Veterinarians and the Veterinary Medical Services in the United States" study sponsor, 1
  Job Bank of, 3, 105
American Veterinary Medical Foundation, ClientLink video training program of, 54
Ancillary services, **99–103**
  boarding, 11, 99–100
  expanded patient services, 102–103
  grooming, 100–102
  pet boutiques, 101–102
  photography, 101–102
Anesthesia, blood screening prior to, 119
Animal caretakers, 31
Animal Care Training, 54
Annual life-cycle consultations, 36, 38, 120
Anthrozoos, 6–7
Appointment hours, 9, 45
  evening hours, 55, 113, 114, 117
  expansion of, 113–114, 117
  for senior-citizen clients, 115
  24-hours, 122–123
  weekend, 55, 114, 117
Appraisal interview, 141
Appraisals, of staff performance, 53, 96, 109, 145
Aprons, use during grooming, 77–78
Assets, separation from resources, 128
Associates, 5, 105–106
  computer literacy of, 105
  fringe benefits for, 105
  impact on client access scheduling, 107, 128
  income and wages of, 2, 5, 32, 98
  integration into healthcare delivery team, 106
  management role of, 95
  nonmonetary rewards for, 131
  productivity of, 3, 95–96
  recruitment of, 105

163

Index

Association dues, as benefit, 98
Attitude
  of staff members, 43–44, 46
  of the workplace, 95
Attorneys, corporate, 6, 18
Authority, 141
Average client transaction (ACT), 14, 141
AVMA. *See* American Veterinary Medical Association

Balanced lifestyle, 2, 131–132
Balance sheets, 17
Bankers, personal business, 18
Bank loans
  personal guarantees for, 109
  for purchase of veterinary hospitals, 14
Bathing, protective clothing for, 77–78
Bathing services, 99, 100
Bed and breakfast, for cats and dogs, 100
Behavior
  definition of, 141
  of staff, 46
  modification of, 51–52
Behavior management center, 102
Belize, 47
Benchmarking, 58–59, 141
Benefits
  for new associates, 105
  for staff, 97–98
Bites, as recordable workplace accidents, 80–81
Blame, avoidance of, 1
Bloodborne Pathogens Standard, 85, 86, 88–89
Blood screening, preanesthetic, 119
Boarding services, 12, 31
  as day care, 102
Body language, 141
Bonding, client-veterinarian, 40–41, 128
Bookkeeping systems, computer-based, 26
Boredom, avoidance of, 47
Boutiques, pet, 101–102
Boy Scouts of America, 47
Brain-picking, 58
Brainstorming, 10, 46, 49–50, 142
Brochures, 114, 125
Budgeting/budgets
  definition of, 142
  for new practices, 16–19
  program-based, 16–17, 128, 146
Building the Successful Veterinary Practice: Innovation and Creativity, Vol. 3 (Catanzaro), 44

Building the Successful Veterinary Practice: Programs and Procedures, Vol. 2 (Catanzaro), 17, 92, 93
Business image, effect of incorporation on, 110
Business plan, 9
Business skills, of veterinarians, 5–6
Business start-up checklist, 9–10
Business team, 17
"Buzz phrases," 57

"Camps," for dog field trial areas, 100
Cardiac evaluations, 120
Cardiopulmonary resuscitation (CPR), 89
Caring, 132
Catchment areas, 12–13, 142
Cat food, sale of, 117–118
Cats
  boarding space requirements for, 99
  declawing of, 120
CD-ROM
  Material Safety Data Sheets on, 75, 76
  OSHA regulations on, 72–73
Centers for Disease Control (CDC), 118
Certified Veterinary Practice Managers, 98, 108
Chamber of Commerce, 14, 29, 36
Chemical Hazard Communication Program, 30
Chemicals, flushing from eyes, 77
"Chute mentality," 6
Civic affairs. *See also* Community organizations
  veterinarians' participation in, 40
Client(s), 113–114
  differentiated from customers, 113
  location of, 12
  new, 121
    acquisition of, 36
    first office visit with, 37
    "goody bags" for, 39–40
    preferred, 36
    price shopping by, 114–115
    reduced flow of, 115
    "two-yes" options for, 2, 37
    types of, 35
    walk-ins, 116
    "yes-no" options for, 37
Client access, expansion of, 107, 115, 128
Client-centered practice, 10, 107
Client/customer services, **113–126**
Client demand, effect on appointment hours, 113

Client education, 102, 111
  following price increases, 116
  Internet-based, 27
ClientLink (video training program), 54
Client transactions
  number per month
    average, 14, 141
      as indicator of need for staff expansion, 107
      at peak performance, 107, 116, 132
Client-veterinarian bonding, 37, 40–41, 128
Clinical skills, deficits in, 5–6
Coaching, of new associates, 106
Code of Federal Regulations, 99
Commitment, 142
Communication method, 142
Communication process, 142
Community organizations
  donations to, 122
  as support network, 50
  veterinarians' support of, 6, 122
Community pet-related causes, veterinarians' participation in, 39
Compassionate care, 3
Compensation. *See also* Wages; W-2 compensation package
  for groomers, 100
  for new associates, 105
Competency, of staff members, 32–33, 43, 45, 51
Competitors, unprofessional behavior by, 39
Competiveness, relationship to appointment hours, 122–123
Computer literacy, of new associates, 105
Computers, 19–29. *See also* Internet
  bookkeeping applications of, 26
  implication for client-veterinarian relationship, 41
  leasing of, 22–25
  software for, 22, 25–26, 76
  use in staff training, 64
  training in use of, 21–22, 28
Condos, for cats, 99
Consultations, annual life-cycle, 36, 38, 120
Consulting firms/teams, 6, 18
Continuing education
  Internet-based, 28
  for staff, 28, 33, 108
Continuous quality improvement (CQI), 48, 96, 108, 142
Contracts
  for computer leasing, 23–25
  negotiation of, 15, 23

Controlled substances, 89–91
Core values, 10, 11, 17, 106, 133, 142
Corporate attorneys, 18
Corporate papers, registration of, 9
Corporation. *See also* Incorporation
  limited liabillity corporation (LLC), 110, 128
Correspondence training, of staff, 64–65
Coupons, 37, 115
CQI (continuous quality improvement), 46, 48, 108, 142
Creativity
  blockage of, 50
  critical elements of, 58
  of staff members, 45–46, 48–50
Credit cards, 14
Credit risk, of veterinarians, 14
Curb cut locations, for veterinary practices, 12
"Current and Future Market for Veterinarians and the Veterinary Medical Services in the United States," 1–7
Customers, differentiated from clients, 113

Darwin, Charles, 58
Day care, 102
Decision making
  definition of, 142
  support network for, 50
Declawing, of cats, 120
Delegation, of responsibility or obligations, 106, 142
Delta Society, 102
Dental hygiene specialists, 107, 108
Deworming, 118
Dips, safety precautions for use of, 77–78
Direction-persuasion-coaching approach, in staff orientation training, 53
Disabilities, of staff, 30
Disability insurance, 98
Disciplining, of staff, 51–52
  for refusal to follow safety rules, 78
Discounts, 37, 115. *See also* Coupons
Disposal, of controlled substances, 91
Distance-learning programs, for staff, 43–44, 108
Distributors
  participation in recruitment of new associates, 105
  staff training by, 54
Division of work, 142
Divorce, 131
Dog field trials, "camp" for, 101

Dog food, sale of, 117–118
Donations, 122
Drinking, in hazardous areas, 78–79
Drop-off privileges, for clients, 113, 114, 128
Drop-out rate, in veterinary medicine, 132
Drugs
  as controlled substances, 89–91
  delayed payment plans for, 14
  inventory costs of, 48
  refill tracking systems for, 92

Eating, in hazardous areas, 78–79
Edison, Thomas, 38
Effectiveness, 132–133
Efficacy, 132–133
Efficiency, 132–133
E-mail, 27
Emergency notification posters, 84–85
Emergency situations, 84–89
Employee-centered supervision, 142
Employee counseling, 143
Employees. *See* Staff
Employee turnover, 143
Employment brokerages, veterinary-specific, 5, 95
Endorsements, 46
Environmental regulations. *See* Occupational Safety and Health Administration (OSHA)
Equine practices, 11, 14, 124
Equipment
  diagnostic, payment for, 120
  for new veterinary practices, 15, 29–30
Equipment trusts,
Evacuation, of animals, in emergencies, 85–86
Excellence, internal focus of, 57
Exhaust, differentiated from ventilation, 79
Exits, emergency, 87
Expanded patient services, 102–103
Expansion, of healthcare delivery team, 106–110
Externship programs, as source of new associates, 105
Eyewashes, 76–77

Facilitating, 143
Failure, fear of, 47
Family, of veterinarians, 131
"Fat farms," 102
Faucets, use in eye flushing, 77
Fax transmissions, cost of, 18–19

Fecal examinations, 76, 118
Feedback, 143
Fees/fee schedules. *See also* Pricing, of services
  reasonable, 110–111
  of women veterinarians, 2–3
Financial advice/planning, 6. *See also* Budgeting/budgets; Succession planning
Financing, of new practices, 14–15
Fire extinguishers, 86–87
Firing, of staff, 33–34
  for refusal to follow safety procedures, 77–78
First-aid kits, 89
"First death" partner insurance, 98
Five-exposure rule, 125
Flashlights, as emergency lights, 88
Flexibility, absolute rigid, 141
Flexible scheduling, 45, 105
Fluoroscopy procedures, safety procedures for,
Followup, in marketing of practice, 115
Foreign bodies, ocular, eyewashes for, 77
Fortune 500 companies, 18, 58
Franklin, Benjamin, 58
Free association, of ideas, 143
Free-standing facilities, 14, 15–16
Friends, 131
Fringe benefits. *See* Benefits
Full time equivalent (FTE) doctor computations, 13, 121

Glossary, **141–147**
Goals, written, 58
Goal setting, for new practices, 9
Goggles, safety, 77–78
"Goody bags," for new clients, 39–40
"Grapevine" (information network), 143
"Gripe sessions," meetings as, 64
Grooming, protective clothing and goggles for, 77–78
Grooming services, 31, 100
Group dynamics, 143

"Hall of fame," 49
Halo effect, 143
Hazardous medical waste, 83–84
Healthcare
  definition of, 143
  quality of, 2
Healthcare delivery
  inefficiency of, 4

Healthcare delivery *(cont.)*
  new ideas for, 56
  quality of, 2
  social contract in, 113, 116–117
Healthcare delivery team
  expansion of, 106–110
  integration of new associates into, 106
Healthcare programs, 10
Health insurance
  for pets, 45, 102
  for veterinarian and staff, 105
Health regulations. *See* Occupational Safety and Health Administration (OSHA) regulations
HEAP (history, evaluation, assessment, plan) approach, to medical record organization, 143
Heartworm, 118
Heller, Steve, 57
Help-wanted ads, 44
Hiring teams, 32, 43
History, evaluation, assessment, plan (HEAP) approach, to medical record organization, 143
Home visits, 102
Hoses, use for eye flushing, 77
Hospital administrators, 98. *See also* Managers
Hospitals
  construction costs of, 15, 99
  financing of, 14–15
Hospital safety manuals, 74
Hotels, for pets, 100
Humane Society, practice linkages with, 102
Human-relations management, 143
Human resources. *See* Staff

Idea lotteries, 48
Idea quotas, 48
Ideas
  barriers to, 50
  free association of, 143
Identification (IDs), for pets, 103
Identification numbers, for staff members, 10
Incentives, for staff members, 45–48
Income, 1. *See also* Wages
  annual, 114
  components of, 131
  of first-year practices, 35
  gross, wages as percentage of, 48
  net, 56
  effect of price increases on, 116

Income *(cont.)*
  relationship to productivity, 3
  stagnation of, 5
  of women veterinarians, 1–2
Income statements, 17
Incorporation, 9, 109–110
Indifference, as mediocrity cause, 144
Infinity model, of leadership and management, 144
Inner strength, 144
Innovation, 45–46, 48–50, 56
Insecticide application, use of protective equipment during, 77–78
In-service training, 53–54
Insurance, 10. *See also* Health insurance
Internet, 26–29. *See also* Web sites
  certified veterinary technician programs on, 44
  marketing on, 29
  OSHA regulations on, 73
  practice consultant selection guidelines on, 18
  use in recruitment of new associates, 105
  staff use policy for, 28
  use in recruitment and training of staff, 28
  veterinary safety program information on, 27
Internship programs, as source of new associates, 105
Interviewing, of job applicants,
Interviews, appraisal, 141
Intravenous fluids, use during surgery, 119–120
Inventories
  of controlled substances, 89–91
  cost reduction for, 48
Inventory management teams, 48

Jargon, 57, 144
Job aids, 144
Job competency, of staff members, 32–33, 43, 45
Job position description, for staff members, 44–45, 52
Job roles, 144
Job sharing, 97
Journal of the American Veterinary Medical Association, 1
Journals, daily, 58
Jung, Carl, 58

Kal Kan Foods, Inc., 52
Ketamine hydrochloride abuse, 131

Kitten carrier classes, 103
Knowledge brokering, 57
Kroc, Ray, 11

Labor laws, 10. *See also* Occupational Safety and Health Administration (OSHA) regulations
Land, purchase of, 15
Landscaping, 16
Larval migrans, 118
Laser surgery, 120
Lawsuits, 92–93
Leader, definition of, 144
Leadership
  of healthcare delivery team, 128–129
  infinity model of, 144
  operational, 127
  in staff training, 61–62
  as succession planning issue, 127, 128–129
Leadership teams, 106
Leaseholds, 15, 16
Leases
  for computers, 22–25
  defaults on, 109
Legal issues
  affecting new practices, 9–10
  lawsuits, 92–93
  liability, 2, 79–80, 109–110
  in succession planning, 127–129
Leisure time activities, 131
Lending library, 103
Letters of admonishment, 78
Liability
  effect of incorporation on, 2, 109–110
  for work-related accidents, 79–80
Licenses, for new practices, 9
Licensing fees, payment of, as job benefit, 98
Life-cycle consultations, annual, 36, 38, 120
Lifestyle
  balanced, 2, 131–132
  creativity as, 50
Lights, emergency, 88
Limited liability partnership (LLP), 110, 128
Limited liabillity corporation (LLC), 110, 128
Listening, active, 141
Litigation, 92–93
Litigious, definition of, 144
LLC (limited liabillity corporation), 110, 128
LLP (limited liability partnership), 110, 128

Loans
  defaults on, 109
  for purchase of veterinary hospitals, 14, 15
Location
  of clients, 12
  of veterinary practices, 9
    as basis for clients' selection of veterinarians, 36
  elements of, 121
  of new practices, 12–14
Logos, 101, 124–125

Malpractice, 92–93
Management
  human-relations, 143
  "millennium," 56–59
  by nonowner veterinarians, 95
  open-book, 48
  "sounds bites for success" in, **135–139**
  total quality (TQM), 147
Management bookkeeping, 26
Management development, 144
Managers
  Certified Veterinary Hospital, 98, 108
  definition of, 144
  of emergency plans, 85
Manuals
  computer users,' 21
  hospital safety, 74
  policy, 52
  for staff training, 52
Marketing, 121–126. *See also* Advertising
  on the Internet, 29
  media use in, 115
  for new clients, 114–115
  plan for, 9
  after price increases, 116
  staff's role in, 40
Master problem list, 92
Material Safety Data Sheets (MSDS), 27, 75–76
Medical records
  format of, 92–93
  length of retention of, 93
  organization of
    HEAP (history, evaluation, assessment, plan) approach to, 143
    SOAP (subjective, objective, assessment, plan) approach to, 93, 146
Medical waste, hazardous, 83–84
Medication refill tracking system, 92

Mediocrity, in healthcare, 111
Meetings
 formal, 64
 as "gripe sessions," 64
 as staff training method, 64, 66, 67–69
 successful, guidelines for, 67–68
 timing of, 67, 68, 69
 videotaping of, 66
Memos, use in staff training, 66–67
Mentors/mentoring, 129
 definition of, 144
 of new associates, 106
 in staff training, 54
Metcalfe, Jack, 47
Millennium management, 56–59
Mind maps, 46, 49, 58
Minors, as staff members, X-ray machine use by, 83
Mission focus, 11
Modeling, definition of, 144
"Monday Morning Memo," 65
Motivation
 definition of, 144
 of staff members, 45–48

Name, of practice, 9
Name recognition, 123
Needles, as hazardous medical waste, 84
Needlestick injuries, 81–82
Network of Animal Health (NOAH), 30
New practices, **9–41**
 advertising of, 9, 10, 36
 budget of, 16–19
 business start-up checklist for, 9–10
 clients of, 35–41
 computerization of, 19–29
 equipment and inventory of, 29–30
 financing of, 14–15
 first-year transactions of, 35
 income of, 35
 leasehold versus free-standing, 15–16
 location of, 12–14
 minimum essential services of, 37–38
 safety requirements for, 30–31
 staffing of, 31–34
Newsletters, 115
Newspaper articles, as publicity source for new practices, 36
Newspapers, help-wanted ads in, 44
NOAH (Network of Animal Health), 30
Nonattendance, by staff, at training sessions, 69
North American Compendiums, Inc., 76

Northwest Veterinary Managers Association, 7
Notes, use in staff training, 66–67
Nurses
 client education and followup responsibilities of,
 home visits by, 102
 input, 55, 107
 outpatient, 34, 107
Nurses aides, as veterinary staff members, 43
Nursing telephone outreach, 108
Nutritional centers, 101
Nutritional counseling/counselors, 48, 108, 118

Objectives, definition of, 145
Occupational Safety and Health Administration (OSHA), inspection of veterinary practices by, 71–72
Occupational Safety and Health Administration (OSHA) regulations, 71–89
 available on the Internet, 73
 Bloodborne Pathogens Standard, 85, 86, 88–89
 compliance with, 73
 for emergency plans, 84–89
 Form 200 of, 80
 implementation plans for, 73–75
 Material Safety Data Sheets for, 27, 75–76
 violations of, fines for, 72
Office displays, 101
"Ogre," 145
Older pets, respite care for, 102
One-on-one style, of staff training, 64–65
On-the-job style, of staff training, 64
Open-book management, 48
Orientation training. *See* Training and orientation
Orthopedic Foundation for Animals (OFA) certification, 102
OSHA. *See* Occupational Safety and Health Administration
Outcome excellence, 106
Outer strength, 145
Overhead, monthly, 110

Pain management, 118–119
Paraprofessionals. *See* Staff
Parasite prevention and control center/counseling, 102, 107

Participation, 145
Partners. *See also* Associates
    as practice leaders, 127
Partnership, limited liability partnership (LLP), 110, 128
Partnership papers, registration of, 9
Patient advocacy, 10, 31, 46, 145
Patient data sheet, 92
Peace of mind, of clients, as veterinary practice commodity, 2, 117, 118, 133
Peer-to-peer message boards, 27
PEN-HIP certification, 102
Performance appraisals, 53, 96, 109, 145
Performance planning, 53
Permits, for new practices, 9
Personal calling, veterinary practice as, 11, 132
Personal-days account, 98
Personality, 145
Personal life. *See* Lifestyle
Personal relationships, 131, 132
Personnel manuals. *See* Policy manuals
Pet boutiques, 101–102
Pet-center complex, 16
Pet food, sale of, 117–118
Pet health insurance, 102
Pet hotels, 100
Pet Partner Program, 102
Pet population
    implication for siting of new practices, 13–14
    stabilization of, 56
Pet population control clinics, 114
Pet resorts, 99–100
Pets by Prescription, 102
Pfizer, 6–7
Photography services, 101
Physician extenders, 4. *See also* Veterinary extenders
"Piercing the corporate veil," 109
Planning
    performance, 53
    succession, **127–129**
    definition of, 146
Policies, definition of, 145
Policy manuals, 52
Population control clinics, 114
Practice
    name of, 9
    new. *See* New practices
    nontraditional, 4
    sale of. *See* Succession planning
Practice brochures, 114, 125

Practice owner, definition of, 145
Practice ownership, succession planning for, **127–129**, 146
Practice programs, staff support for, 46–47
Practice training manuals, 52
Prescription writing, Drug Enforcement Agency regulations for, 91
Price-centered practices, 37
Price shopping, by clients, 114–115
Pricing, of services, 2, 110–111, 114–115.
    See also Coupons; Discounts
    excessive, 2, 110–111
Pride, of veterinary staff, 2, 111
PRIDE mnemonic, for core values of veterinary practice, 11
Proactive, definition of, 145
Problem solving. *See also* Creativity; Innovation
    definition of, 145
Procedures, definition of, 145
Productivity
    of associates, 3, 95–96
    definition of, 146
    relationship to income, 3
    of staff members, 45
Product literature, 114–115
Professional environment, for staff members, 45
Profitable programs, 11–12
Program-based budgets, 16–17, 128, 146
Progress notes, 93
Promotional displays, 122
Promotional offers, 101. *See also* Coupons; Discounts
Protective equipment
    for application of dips or shampoos, 77–78
    for X-ray machine use, 82
Protocols, for services, staff members' adherence to,
Publicity, for new practices, 36. *See also* Advertising
Puppy classes, 102
"Puppy passports," 103
Purpose, definition of, 146

Quality, of healthcare, 2
    relationship to fees, 111
Quality, value, service, and cleanliness (Q-V-S-C) core values, 11
Quality assurance, 146
Quality control, 146
Quality improvement, 33

Quality of life, 2, 131–132
QuickBooks, 17–18, 26
Quick fix, 146
Q-V-S-C (quality, value, service, and cleanliness) core values, 11

Rabies vaccination, pre-exposure, of staff, 84
Radiation Safety Program, 30
Rand, Paul, 57
Reading list, **159–162**
Real estate investments, 129
Receptionists, 31, 32–33, 34
  role in marketing of practice, 40
  training and orientation checklist for, 149–153
Recognition, of staff members' creativity, 48–49
Recommendations, as source of new clients, 36, 37, 38
Recovered client programs, 37, 107
Recovered patient programs, 107
Recruitment
  of associates, 105
  of staff, 33, 43–45
Referrals
  to specialty practices, 121
  word-of-mouth, 36, 37, 38
Regular resale area, 101
Regulations, **71–93**. See also Occupational Safety and Health Administration (OSHA) regulations
  for controlled substances, 89–91
  definition of, 146
Remedial training, of staff, 63
Reminder cards, 38, 125
Resale area, regular, 101
Research, Internet use in, 27
Resorts, for pets, 56, 99–100
Resources, separation from assets, 128
Respect, responsibility, and recognition (Three Rs), of staff employment, 45, 46
Respite care, 103
Responsibility
  definition of, 146
  delegation of, 106, 142
  of new associates, 106
Retirement planning, 98, 129
Rights, of the employed, **95–98**
Right to Know Program, 30
R. K. House & Associates, Ltd, 6
Runs, size of, 99

Safety programs, key elements of, 30–31
Safety regulations. See also Occupational Safety and Health Administration (OSHA) regulations
  available on the Internet, 27, 73
Satisfaction, definition of, 146
Savings, for retirement, 98, 129
"Schedule the hospital," 55
Scheduling
  of appointment hours, 55
  flexible, 45, 105
  high-density, 3, 4, 45, 96
  linear, 3, 4, 96, 107
  of staff training, 65–66
Scratches, as recordable workplace accidents, 80–81
"Sell the sizzle," 46–47
Senior citizens, as clients, 115, 125–126
Senior pet classes, 102
Separation, of assets and resources, 128
Service Corps of Retired Executives, 9
Shampoos, safety precautions for use of, 77–78
Sharps, as hazardous medical waste, 84
Shaw, George Bernard, 57
Signature Series Monographs, 93, 118
Signs,
  for new practices, 36
  use in staff training, 66–67
  visibility of, 12, 121
Signs, 121
  for emergency exits, 87
Small Business Administration, 9
SOAP (subjective, objective, assessment, plan) approach, to medical record organization, 93, 146
Social contract, in healthcare delivery, 113, 116–117
Software, 25–26, 76
Specialists, board-certified, wages of, 32
Specialty practices, 1–2, 31, 32, 121
Staff, **43–59**. See also Animal caretakers; Nurses; Veterinary technicians
  attitude of, 43–44
  benefits for, 97–98
  competency of, 32–33, 43, 45, 51
  continuing education for, 28, 33, 108
  counseling of, 143
  creativity and innovation of, 45–46, 48–50
  disabilities of, 30
  disciplining of, 51–52
    for refusal to follow safety rules, 78

Staff *(cont.)*
  emergency life-saving assistance by, 89
  firing of, 33–34, 77–78
  identification numbers for, 10
  information "grapevines" of, 143
  legal liability of, 109–110
  marketing of practice by, 40
  minors as, X-ray macine use by, 83
  motivation versus incentives for, 45–48
  of new practices, 31–34
  nonattendance at training sessions, 69
  number of, 123
    implication for OSHA regulations, 71
  part-time, benefits for, 97
  performance appraisals of, 53, 96, 109, 145
  pet health insurance benefit for, 45, 98, 102
  policy manuals for, 52
  pre-exposure rabies vaccinations of, 84
  pride of, 2, 111
  as primary patient care providers, 3
  recruitment of, 33, 43–45
  replacement cost for, 7
  respect, responsibility, and recognition for, 45, 46
  response to stress, 34
  retention of, 34
  tardiness of, 51
  titles of, 34
  training and orientation of, **61–69**
    checklists for, **145–158**
    in use of computer systems, 20, 21–22, 28
    in safety implementation plans, 74–75, 85
    scheduling of, 65–66
    timing of, 62–63
    types of, 63–65
  turnover of, 61, 143
  wages of, 31–32, 48
    inadequate, 7
    pay differentials for evening or weekend work time, 117
    raises in, 31, 132
Staff ratio, paraprofessional/veterinarian, 107
Standards of practice, staff members' adherence to, 53
Stasis, 146
State of Nevada Veterinary Board, 119
Store-front practices, 15, 16
Strategic foresight, 56

Strategic positioning, of new practices, 9
Strength, inner and outer, 144
Stress, 34, 146
"Stupid idea" week contest, 49
Subjective, objective, assessment, plan (SOAP) approach, to medical record organization, 93, 146
Substance abuse, by veterinarians, 131
Success, secret to, 57
Succession planning, **127–129**, 146
Supervision, employee-centered, 94
Supervisor, definition of, 147
Supplies. *See also* Distributors; Vendors
  ordering of, on the Internet, 27
Support networks, 50
Surgery, intravenous fluid use during, 119–120
Synergy, definition of, 147
System, definition of, 147

Tardiness, of staff members, 51
Tax accounting, 26
Tax issues
  corporate structure, 110, 128
  leasing of computers, 22
Teaching hospitals, veterinary, linear scheduling approach of, 4
Team fit, of staff members, 43
Teeth, grading of, 102
Telephone bills, 18–19
Telephone etiquette, "on-hold" messages, 122
Telephone outreach, 108
Telephone screening, of job applicants, 44
Terminology. *See also* Glossary; Jargon
  of staff positions, 34
  of veterinary practice in the new millennium, 57
Tertiary care
  linear scheduling approach in, 4
  as new veterinary graduates' focus, 10
Thoracic wall cardiac monitors, 120
Three Rs (respect, responsibility, and recognition), of staff employment, 45, 46
Time, monetary value of, 96–97
Timing. *See also* Scheduling
  of meetings, 68, 69
  of staff training, 69
Total quality management (TQM), 147
TQS/TMS (total quality service/total management service), 147
Trademarks, 9

Training and orientation
  of new associates,
  of staff, **61–69**
    checklists for, **149–158**
    in use of computer systems, 20, 21–22, 28
    in safety implementation plans, 74–75, 85
    scheduling of, 65–66
    timing of, 62–63
    types of, 63–65
Training manuals, 52
Transactions. *See* Client transactions
Travel, by clients, 39–40
Trivia, administration, 141
"Two-fur-one" programs, 115
"Two-yes" option, for veterinary services, 2, 37

U. S. Drug Enforcement Agency
  compliance with, 89–91
  licensure by, 98
U. S. Government Printing Office, 72–73
Unity of direction, 147

Vacation/holiday pay, 98
Vaccination clinics, 114
Vaccinations, as income source, 56
Values
  core, 10, 11, 17, 106, 133, 142
  definition of, 147
VECCS (Veterinary Emergency and Critical Care Society), 118
Vedco (www.vedco.com), 76
Vehicles, financing of, 14
Vendors
  of computer systems, 19, 20–21, 22, 23–25
  staff training by, 54
Ventilation, differentiated from exhaust, 79
Veterinarians. *See also* Associates
  new graduates
    clinical skills of, 5–6
    drop-out rate of, 132
    job offers to, 3
    practice choices of, 5
    wages of, 2, 5
    work-week length of, 2, 3
  private-practice, shortage of, 4–5
  women, 2–3
Veterinary Compendium, 118
Veterinary Consultant Network, 18

Veterinary Emergency and Critical Care Society (VECCS), 118
Veterinary extenders, 4, 45, 106–107
Veterinary Hospital Managers Association, 98, 108
Veterinary Information Network (www.vin.com), 27
Veterinary Safety and Health Digest, 31
Veterinary Support Network (www.vspn.org), 27
Veterinary technician degree, as job fringe benefit, 44
Veterinary technician programs, Internet-based, 44
Veterinary technicians, 34. *See also* Nurses; Veterinary extenders
  client-centered, 31
  drop-out rate of, 132
  restricted roles of, 7
  training and orientation checklist for, 153–158
Vicarious liability, 109
Videotaping, of meetings, 66
Video training programs, for staff members, 64
  in computer training, 21
Vinci, Leonardo da, 58
VIP resort suites, for pets, 56

W. A. Butler (www.wabutler.com), 76
Wages, 2, 5
  of associates, 25, 32, 98
  as percentage of gross income, 48
  of staff, 31–32, 48
    for evening or weekend work time, 117
  inadequate, 7
  raises in, 31, 132
Walk-in clients, 116
Web sites
  of Chambers of Commerce, 29, 36
  Material Safety Data Sheets on, 27
  for veterinary practices, 28–29
We CARE mneumonic, for core values in veterinary care, 11
Weight loss programs, for pets, 102
Welcome Wagon programs, 123–124
Wellness checklist, 92
Wellness programs, 10, 11–12, 102, 117–120
Windows, as emergency exits, 87
Windows-based software, 25
Women, as veterinarians, 2–3

Index

Woolf, Virginia, 58
Word-of-mouth promotion, of new practices, 36, 37, 38
Work, definition of, 147
Workers' compensation, 79, 98
Work life, quality of, 146. *See also* Balanced lifestyle
Work week, 2, 3
W-2 compensation package, 31–32, 133

X-ray machines
   location of, 83
   safety regulations for, 82–84
   300mA, 30

Yellow Pages, 36, 121
"Yes-no" option, for veterinary services, 37

Zoning laws, 9, 12, 16